A Place to Go

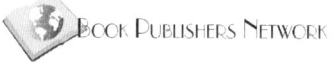

MAUREEN TAYLOR

BOOK PUBLISHERS NETWORK

Book Publishers Network
P.O. Box 2256
Bothell • WA • 98041
PH • 425-483-3040
www.bookpublishersnetwork.com

10 9 8 7 6 5 4 3 2 1

Printed in the United States of America

LCCN 2008906443
ISBN10 1-887542-88-4
ISBN13 978-1-887542-88-3

Proofreader: Julie Scandora
Cover Designer: Laura Zugzda
Typographer: Stephanie Martindale

❦ Foreword ❦

A *Place to Go*, by Maureen Taylor, chronicles the trials and
tribulations of the diagnosis and treatment of connective tissue
diseases, and specifically scleroderma, and the importance of personal
stress in causing and hampering the recovery of patients with
connective tissue disease. Although Maureen may have benefited from
the prescribed medical treatments that she received, she played a large
role in researching and carrying out alternative and natural medical
treatments such as macrobiotics, magnetics, T'ai Chi, and yoga that
seemed to take her initial response to prescribed medications and
turn it into a full remission with disappearance of all her clinical signs
of scleroderma and reduction of her antinuclear antibody testing to
insignificant levels.

Since Maureen made the stunning defeat of her illness public,
researchers at Harvard have reported some therapeutic responses to
minocycline (a first cousin to doxycyline), and researchers at Johns
Hopkins and elsewhere have begun to see responses to CeliCept, a
drug for patients with transplanted organs, and Amevive, a biologic
drug for psoriasis giving hope that a cure for scleroderma may be on
the horizon. Maureen's regimen is considerably less toxic than strong

immunomodular drugs, and all physicians, patients, and investigators need to pay attention to her extraordinary contribution.

Hal Whitman MD FACP FACR
Rheumatology
Summit Medical Group
Summit, New Jersey
and
The Hospital for Special Surgery
New York

❦ Preface ❦

Dealing with scleroderma was a journey home to my inner self. Each step I took in my healing removed one more layer on the outside to bring me closer to who and what I am.

I am indebted to Dr. Hal Whitman as my champion throughout my journey. Along the way, I tried healing methods within both the traditional realm as well as the alternative. Regardless of the ones I chose, Dr. Whitman always supported my efforts. He understood my disease, he knew its path of destruction, and he provided the means for me to find relief from almost constant pain.

Those moments when I had no pain – or at least found the pain lessening where, theretofore, it had only increased – allowed me to assess what was happening to me. Before my pain had so overwhelmed me that I could do little more than merely exist. I'd had no room for healing, only for maintaining the basics of my life.

My journey took me to almost every healing modality that exists. Serendipity seemed to carry me from one method to the next. I would meet just the right person or note a certain article in the newspaper. And what always guided me was my intuition. I was traveling where no others had gone before. The expected, the *guaranteed*, result of my disease was a disfiguring death in the near-term. My inner feeling about whether or not to go with one promising method – and how extensively to use it – was all I had; no one else could guide me. Dr. Whitman gave me the support I so needed, but I was the one making these decisions.

As much as each step I took – each change I embraced – seemed to stall scleroderma and then reverse it, my inner journey was what truly healed me. As I met the demons of my past and made peace with them, I created the inner space for well-being.

These two elements – using my intuition and remaining in peace with myself and all around me – are the foundation to my healing.

And so, I cannot give a formula for anyone else's healing. Each one must find his or her own path. I show how I healed myself that others be inspired and know *miracles are possible*. But the specific steps others must take are their own.

This I do know is true for all on the journey chosen: as we heal ourselves within, we heal without.

May peace be always with you.

✖ Prologue ✖

Until that moment, my body – and the secrets it had kept hidden from me – had been a frustrating and frightening mystery, one that haunted my every waking hour yet revealed itself only partially. In the alien features of the woman staring back at me in the mirror. In my disfigured face, hard as stone and cold to the touch. In the shortness of my breath, the numbness in my head, the swelling in my feet. In the surreal dreamscape I faced every night when I closed my eyes and tried in vain to sleep the sleep of the living.

I was dying. Part of me had known as much for weeks. But until that moment – a muggy August day in 1988 – I had worn my ignorance reluctantly but effectively, like a protective charm. What I didn't know couldn't kill me. Could it?

Dr. Hal Whitman stared back at me without speaking. Blond, nearly six and a half feet tall, he looked like a younger version of the late-night television comedian David Letterman, minus the smirk.

Dr. Whitman was deadpan all right, but with no punch line in sight. I recognized his face; I had met him years earlier while he had been a house doctor and I a private duty nurse at New York Hospital in Manhattan. He didn't recognize me – only the disease that inhabited my body. He had his white coat on and his hands stuffed into his pockets, and he was standing in the doorway staring at me, still not speaking. His shoebox of an office, a modest drive from my home in Wayne, New Jersey, was barely big enough to house a waiting area and the examination room. His nurse, an efficient woman in her sixties with graying hair, protected him like a mother hen guarding one of her chicks.

When he finally spoke, it wasn't to say hello or to introduce himself. He spoke directly to the mystery, the ghastly shell of my former self I had become. "How long have you been like this?" he asked.

"Oh," I said, momentarily taken aback, "for quite a while."

He paused once again, and then walked toward me and took my swollen hands in his. After examining them, he asked me to squeeze his index finger. He must have known already that I couldn't possibly close my hands, much less apply pressure to his index finger. The swelling in my hands had rendered them just shy of useless. I struggled to drive, often dropped things, and had difficulty accomplishing the simplest of tasks. I could hardly even walk anymore, because my skin from the top of my head to the soles of my swollen feet had hardened unmercifully. He continued to inspect the skin on my hands, eyeing the varying shades of blue and purple and white, and then moved his examination to the Formica-hard skin covering my face, which he tried in vain to pinch.

He finally looked up at me and announced matter-of-factly, "You have scleroderma, and from what I can see, it's quite advanced."

Finally, after two years of confusion and fear, I knew what was stalking me. I had seen countless specialists and come up empty each time. I had pursued every potential lead and had even tried to research on my own the roots of my failing health, only to circle but never penetrate the mystery. I had endured the scorn of many, including my husband, who had informed me that the sickness I felt in my bones was all in my head. And more than once I had felt alone – utterly alone – with whatever it was that was slowly stealing my life. Could anyone name my pain?

Dr. Whitman had done so, definitively and decisively. And, as he would on numerous occasions over the course of the next seven years, he indulged me with a thorough explanation.

"Scleroderma is a disease that makes you produce too much collagen," he told me. "The connective tissue in your body – in your skin, your lungs, your heart, your kidneys – eventually hardens. Scleroderma – it's also called systemic sclerosis when it affects the whole body – is classified as an autoimmune disease. We don't know what causes it, and we don't know how to cure it. It's progressive."

And just like that, I knew what had taken over my body – and where it was taking me. I had known deep down that I was dying. Now there was no denying it. I was one of roughly three hundred thousand in the U.S. estimated to have scleroderma, which kills hundreds each year.

The relief of finally being able to name my illness disappeared in the wake of what amounted to a death sentence. I had come this far, only to find out that I had nearly reached the end of my journey. In the months to come – scary, desperate months – I would slowly find the courage to counter death's claim. But for now, the swelling that had incapacitated my feet and hands had spread to my heart. The disfigurement that had turned my fingers into gnarled claws and my face into a ghoulish caricature had reached into my soul. The future – accurately diagnosed and eerily mapped out for me – looked far more frightening than the darkest depths of my imagination.

⊗ 1 ⊗

I remember her fingers, yellow-white and stone-cold to the touch. She would come in out of the cold, having just worked in the garden, and rush to the kitchen sink, where she would dunk her hands in warm water until the color returned to them.

"I have no blood in my fingers," she would say as they thawed. Yellow to purple and finally to pale pink: the pattern is always the same for those plagued by Raynaud's phenomenon, a non-life-threatening but burdensome condition that affects an estimated five to ten percent of the population. My mother suffered its debilitating effects while I was a child growing up in Ireland.

I would, in years to come, become familiar with Raynaud's on a more intimate basis. But for now, it belonged to my mother, whose inscrutable health problems often left her incapacitated and housebound. When she was feeling her worst, she would stay inside for days at a time, sometimes even skipping Mass on Sundays because of head-splitting migraines.

Once, as I left for school, she told me, "I might be dead by the time you get back."

I fretted over her warning all day at school, and when the schoolteacher released us at the end of the day, I came running home, panic-stricken, only to find her in the same condition as when I'd left her in the morning.

I was born in the 1940s toward the tail end of World War II, the third of five children, including my older brothers, Patrick Joseph and Christopher, and my younger sisters, Olive and Evelyn. My father, an only son, was a bachelor for the first forty years of his life, after which he met and married my mother, who was ten years his junior. They settled on a farm in Ireland's rugged interior, conservative country, where hard work was the only currency that counted and the Catholic Church our constant watchdog.

Winters were cold and bleak, often snowy. We walked a mile and a half to a Spartan school, where the heat from the fire in the classroom stove went straight up the chimney and where the teacher cured me of writing left-handed by forcing me to use my right hand when I was just five years old. Physical and abusive, my teacher's methods more than not left me in tears. But no one – not my parents, not my older brothers, not I – ever thought to protest. The church steeple was the highest point on the horizon, and the Catholic hierarchy fostered in our tiny farming community an atmosphere of quiet obedience and tight-lipped sacrifice. Life was hard, and few had the resources to escape.

We did our grocery shopping at the town's only store, but we grew most of our food on the farm. Like our neighbors, our parents were generous people, willing to give whatever they had.

My brothers and sisters and I, meanwhile, gave the only thing of value we possessed: our labor. As soon as we came home from school, we would get to work tackling our daily chores: milking the cows or gathering eggs or working the soil. I can remember planting potatoes while laboring in a frozen March wind, my back aching and my fingers frozen. As soon as the school year came to an end and summer arrived, we were as busy as farmhands, threshing the hay and cutting the grass and weeding the fields and vegetable garden.

Fun came in concentrated and impromptu doses: going to a country dance or sitting around and telling ghost stories in the evening. Perhaps because we knew hard work so well, we also knew how to lose ourselves in the restful moments, to fully experience the good in our lives. We enjoyed talking late into the night, meeting new people, and relishing life's small pleasures.

I was especially close to my father and my older brothers, each of whom looked after me and made me feel safe and protected. My mother, plagued by ill health, did the best she could, despite her circumstances. She had no patience for vanity and, perhaps hoping to cure me of mine, often reminded me that I had an ugly nose.

Her criticism fed my own insecurity, which I would carry with me into adulthood. Not until years later, when a plastic surgeon in the United States told me I had a lovely nose – one that countless of his patients would do anything to have – did I realize my own beauty. Later, after scleroderma had ravaged my face and body, I would call upon my own vanity to help restore that beauty.

As a child, I felt manipulated by my mother's gloomy predictions, her sullenness, and her inability to sustain emotional contact. But now I understand that she battled more than ill health; she was depressed – and had every right to be. She led a hard life, was dealt many emotional blows (including giving birth to a stillborn baby just before me), shouldered a heavy burden (she took care of my grandparents and her father as they aged), and suffered poor nutrition. She received hardly any medical care, which meant her first visit to a doctor during each pregnancy usually came when she delivered. She coped as best she could.

Neither of my parents was outwardly warm, a fact of life that left me scavenging for intimacy. I often took in stray dogs and cats, cuddling with them and putting my head up to their faces and feeling their warmth, even letting them kiss me. I would sneak a puppy or a kitten into the house to sleep with me, hoping my treachery would somehow go unnoticed by my mother. But she would inevitably discover the hideaway and come after the hapless animal with a stick, screaming and flailing her arms as she did.

Perhaps the mere presence of the lovable animal – so dependent upon us and deserving of our affection – only served to remind my mother of an unstated truth in our family: we rarely expressed affection, whether through hugs or kisses or kind words.

The poster child for that emotional defect was my Uncle James, my mother's brother who shared a farmhouse with my grandfather at the time and later lived alone on his own farm. Uncle James always wore a grim expression and had an outlook on life that matched his frown. His strange-looking face and domineering, bossy demeanor alienated him from most people, including the neighborhood children, who made fun of the way he looked. My siblings and I never laughed at his appearance, but it made a formidable impression on all of us. Once, when my sister Evelyn stretched her face into an ugly expression, my mother warned her, "God could leave you like that," which prompted Evelyn to respond, "Is that what happened to Uncle James?"

Uncle James walked on his forefeet and often tripped as he tiptoed. His shirtsleeves hung wide open, and his fingers and hands curled inward like claws. When he bit into a piece of bread, he ate around the crusts because he couldn't chew them. He coughed and gagged when he tried to drink, and his teeth sported gaping spaces between them. I never imagined while watching him struggle at the dinner table that I would one day suffer the same humiliation.

My Grandfather Pat was practically deaf, and we had to shout at him to be heard, but Uncle James coughed every time he tried to raise his voice above a whisper. I can still see my uncle trying to scold my older brother Patrick Joseph, or "Pakie Joe," as we called him, during one visit. Pakie Joe had cut a sally branch, sneaked into the house, and stuck it into the middle of the pot of porridge my grandfather had left simmering over the fire. When Grandfather Pat discovered the branch poking up out of the saucepan like it had grown there, he chased my brother outside, with Uncle James trying to holler after them but choking on his words.

I remember later asking my mother what ailed Uncle James, and she answered that he had contracted polio as a little boy. Only later would I learn that he had likely been suffering from advanced scleroderma, or systemic sclerosis. And with that knowledge, I would look down at my own hands and see gnarled claws and look in the mirror and see a constant, sour frown – the same grim expression of my uncle's. Like him, I would one day gag when I ate or tried to raise my voice. The painful-sounding cough in his chest would eventually echo in mine.

ରେ

Rural Ireland wasn't exactly the place to go for an accurate medical diagnosis in the 1950s. Because we lived so far out in the country and because we had little or no money to spare for medical care, we seldom visited doctors, except for immunizations. I remember suffering my share of health problems growing up, and most were cured the old-fashioned way: by gritting my teeth and outlasting them. Sometimes health care came to us, as when a nurse visited our school and examined us. But even then, that was as far as the care went. When I was diagnosed with anemia after one such visit from a nurse, I was given no treatment.

My lone visit to the country doctor came one morning when I was nine years old and suffering from a severe case of bronchitis. The doctor made weekly visits to the dispensary, so my father dropped me off there on his way to do business at the creamery. The doctor listened with his stethoscope to my chest and prescribed for me bright red cough syrup, and then I took a seat in the front room and waited for my father to return for me. Sitting next to me was the doctor's aunt, a little old lady who rented a room in the house.

The minutes – and eventually the hours – slowly crawled by as I sat there waiting, and I started to feel angry at my mother for not chaperoning me to my first doctor's appointment. That was something she often did: send us kids someplace while she stayed behind. But more than anything, I felt alone – and maybe a little afraid. I couldn't help wishing someone from the family was there to protect and comfort me. My father finally arrived to pick me up at three o'clock, five hours after dropping me off.

I made my first and only childhood trip to the dentist alone, too – or at least without the company of a parent – after Evelyn and I had both complained of toothaches. The dentist at the dispensary, having informed my sister and me that he would be pulling the offending teeth, came at me with an enormous needle. I was terrified but endured the shot of Novocain. As soon as he had finished with the needle, he told us we would need to wait thirty minutes for the Novocain to kick in – plenty of time for us to conspire to escape.

We slipped out the door and ran home. Upon seeing us, Mother told us she never wanted to hear another word about toothaches. The tooth the dentist had planned to pull eventually rotted and fell out on its own.

Overall, I was somewhat of a sickly child, although I didn't realize it at the time. Along with having bronchial asthma, I often experienced mysterious stomach aches that came and went, and I suffered severe migraines, especially on Sundays when we had to fast before communion. Like my mother, I couldn't linger in the summer sun, lest I suffer a red rash on my chest and hands. I rarely felt great, in fact, but I assumed that was normal for everybody.

Then there was the strange and mysterious numbness in my face, which I felt on more than one occasion while drifting off to sleep at night. It felt as if something heavy, like a dinner plate, was resting on my nose and lips. My body felt cold and my face numb, but the sensation never lasted long. Because it seldom came, I never sought help or an explanation.

Later, as a teenager and living at the Marist Convent, where I was a boarding student, I awoke from a deep sleep with severe pain in my side and was rushed in an ambulance to Manor Hamilton Hospital. The doctors there informed me I needed an appendectomy and that they would be performing surgery that night.

My parents, who didn't own a car, were unable to be by my side when the nurses took me into the operating room. I was terrified, especially when the anesthesiologist tried to administer the ether. No one had explained what they were going to do, and I gasped and struggled as they held me down. It felt like I was being smothered.

When I came to, I awoke to a chorus of moaning, courtesy of the other twenty-or-so women on the ward. At about seven o'clock in the morning, the matron of the hospital, a tall, pale Catholic nun, came to see me on her morning rounds. She asked how I felt, and I started to cry and told her I was experiencing a lot of pain.

Instead of comforting me, she put me in my place. "Don't let me hear you talk about pain again," she scolded me. "It's All Soul's Day. Instead of crying, offer your pain up for them."

I felt so stunned that I blurted out, "What do you mean, offer it up for the holy souls? I'm almost one of them myself!"

გე

I had come to the Marist Convent as a boarder student at the tender age of thirteen. The school was run by nuns, all of them highly disciplined in their faith but far more humane than my secular teacher and tormentor back home.

The nuns, ever obedient to the Catholic hierarchy, were a product of the same cloistered world as I was, but while the people back home kept their minds on their work and the trivial meanness of everyday life, the nuns gazed ever heavenward. Under their tutelage, I discovered a wellspring of endurance and an almost magical belief in myself and what fate had in store for me. The troubles so common to today's teenagers – alienation, rebellion, and so on – would have been lost on me. I had snatched a glimpse of myself and what I was worth, and I left the school a young woman with confidence in her future.

As a child brought to Mass each week – from the moment we were born, my brothers and sisters and I were taught by my parents that it was a sin not to go to Mass on Sunday – I had associated religion with confusing rituals and loud priests. (I couldn't understand why the priests were always shouting.) As a boarder student at the convent, I had awoken to a world of compassion. Indeed, as I look back at those days now, I realize the nuns were more spiritual than they were religious.

After graduating and bidding farewell to the nuns, I went on to nursing school in Dublin, where, for four years, I learned the art of nursing while further discovering who I was and who I might someday be. The training was grueling and included three months of night duty each year. During those three months, we still had to attend lectures and prepare for exams every day. We would eat breakfast at night, before we went on duty, and then wolf down dinner in the morning after finishing our shift. By then, I could barely keep my eyes open.

When the Dublin Fire Brigade ambulance brought in a drowning victim one day early in my preliminary training, I had my first on-the-job encounter with death. The unidentified man had fallen into the river and had been pronounced dead at the hospital. One of my duties as a nurse – and one that I dreaded – was to help clean up the body and prepare it for the morgue.

As I cleaned the man, I couldn't help wondering about him. Who was he? What was his story? I was overcome with a morbid sense of curiosity, and for days I fought wave after wave of depression. I lay awake each night, trying to make sense of the unidentified man's death. Who did he have in his life? Was he hungry? Homeless? What happened?

In retrospect, I can't help thinking that inexperienced nurses – barely eighteen and on their own for the first time – should have been provided some sort of support network to help them sort through their feelings after such a traumatic event. But we were expected to bury our emotions, lest they bury us. Of course, emotions like those never disappear. They come back to haunt us later in life, and we struggle to name them or their source. Years later, I would learn to let such pain go. But as a young nurse, I simply swallowed it and tried to move on.

My first experience with death had actually occurred years earlier, when I was about nine years old and my grandfather died on Halloween. He had been my godfather, not to mention my kind-hearted protector. Whenever one of us kids got scolded or spanked, he would come running to save us. He had always played games with us on Halloween, like bobbing for apples. But the Halloween he died marked a transition for me.

We held the wake at our home, since back then in Ireland there were no funeral homes, and our neighbors and friends came to pay their respects. People were in and out of the house all day, and their conversations echoed in my ears. I viewed my grandfather's body lying on the bed and thought he looked like he was sleeping. I then sat in the corner in the kitchen and tried not to cry, but I could feel a lump in my throat the size of an orange. Nobody was crying, though, so I did everything I could to hide my emotions, too. My grandfather had lived a long, full life, but for me, the world seemed to be coming to an end. Nobody had ever talked to me about death, or heaven, or what became of us.

Before I went to sleep that night, I stared at his shoes and realized that I wasn't going to be able to talk to him. The finality of death was overwhelming.

⊙⊙

Sometime toward the end of nursing school, after I had turned twenty-two, I learned to smoke. Soon I was a practicing nurse. But I did not intend to ply my trade in Ireland forever. I was ready for adventure, ready to explore the world. My whole life was ahead of me, it seemed to me. And New York City, where my Aunt Mary and her husband, Mike, lived and ran a neighborhood store, beckoned.

ඥ 2 ඥ

I was Irish, had grown up on a farm, and was only twenty-two at the time. But four years of going to nursing school and working at a busy hospital in Dublin had prepared me for my journey across the Atlantic. Touching down in New York City in 1965 felt like coming home. In fact, I fell in love with the Big Apple from nearly the moment I arrived.

I was following in the footsteps of my older brother Chris, who had moved to New York City a few years earlier to stake out a new life. Chris and his fiancée, plus my Aunt Mary, met me at the airport. Aunt Mary and Mike had graciously offered to put me up in their top-floor three-bedroom apartment in the Inwood neighborhood until I could find a place of my own. Since they were in the middle of getting ready to move to a new place, I slept on the couch in the living room.

Anyone who has experienced the distinct odor of mothballs – that strange, antiseptic smell that invades and pervades – knows that few odors leave a more lasting or evocative impression. To this day, when I think of my aunt's home, I think of mothballs; conversely, the slightest whiff of mothballs makes me think of my aunt's musty apartment. The odor was as powerful as it was omnipresent, and since I was (and still am) madly allergic, I had an immediate and violent reaction.

Chris came to take me out on a whirlwind tour of downtown New York. When I returned to the apartment Aunt Mary wanted to know where we had just been; the only place I could remember because I'd seen so much in one day was Times Square. She gasped, "Jesus, Mary, and Joseph! Do you know what kinds of people go down there?"

I quickly learned that I wasn't allowed to go out alone, that there were certain neighborhoods that were strictly off limits, and that Aunt Mary was going to seriously cramp my style.

I came down with a cold the following evening, no doubt a reaction to the mothballs. But my aunt made her own diagnosis: I had the "grip." She marched me down to the doctor's office, where I was given a flu shot, something she had been insisting I get since my arrival. Oh, God, was I sick after that! It would be some time before the abdominal pain and nausea totally disappeared, and I have a hunch the vaccination had a long-term effect on my immune system.

But Aunt Mary was just getting warmed up. Once she had taken care of my health, she declared that my hair was too long and took me to the barbershop for an unceremonious hack job. I couldn't look in the mirror for days.

A stocky woman in her late sixties with dark bags under her eyes, Aunt Mary was my mother's sister. She had a sharp voice, and she talked constantly – to everyone but her husband. She and Mike had had two children together, including a son who had died quite young, and they had both worked hard all their lives. Now, in the twilight of their years, they seemed to have nothing left to say to each other. Mike would leave early every morning for work without saying goodbye or giving her a hug or kiss – he would just walk out. And when Aunt Mary wanted him to bring home a bagful of groceries, she would call him at their little family grocery store in Brooklyn and simply start in on her list when he answered. "Green beans," she would say, "cauliflower, potatoes." As soon as she had finished her list, she would hang up.

Sometimes the eerie dynamics of their relationship, not to mention Aunt Mary's bossy nature, would get to me. That was when

I would go to my brother Chris for an equal dose of humor and commiseration.

"Just let it go in one ear and out the other," he would tell me.

But I couldn't wait to escape, and my brother, whose fiancée had a little apartment over in Washington Heights, eventually offered their place for me to stay until I could get my own apartment.

৩৫

I was still staying at Aunt Mary's when I landed my first job in America. I had hoped to put my nursing training to good use, but when I found out I needed to take two more courses before I could earn my credentials and that I could only work under temporary certification, I decided to look for other work. I was already making so many adjustments at the time – and I wanted so badly to start supporting myself – that I was willing to take on a temporary job until I had earned my nursing credentials.

So I sneaked out of Aunt Mary's apartment one day and took the subway all the way downtown to the financial district. The hordes of people hurrying along the sidewalks while clutching their briefcases fascinated me, and without knowing the first thing about it, I set out to get a job in an office.

I found myself at 2 Rector Street, at the offices of an engineering firm, and I walked into the lobby, stepped onto the elevator, and asked the man standing next to me, "How do you get a job here?"

The man seemed surprised by my question but directed me to the personnel department, where I met a woman who asked what skills I had to offer.

"I'm a nurse," I answered.

She smiled and said, "Well, we don't have any openings for nurses here, but we have a job available as a file clerk."

I think my naiveté and my straight-forward approach endeared me to her, and I left the building with my first job in America.

Not surprisingly, Aunt Mary threw a fit when I got home. She told me to forget the job and find one in nursing, but I knew I needed to get my bearings first, so I defied her and stayed at the firm, where

I worked as a file clerk while I took the courses I needed in order to earn my nursing certification.

I landed my first professional job a year later at New York City's Saint Elizabeth Hospital. I had actually been there several months before – as a patient – after rushing to the emergency room with severe abdominal pain. I was suffering from an intersucception of the colon, a rare medical occurrence that usually only happens to baby boys in the first six months of their lives. It's easy now to wonder if the condition was a harbinger of things to come. At the time, I thought little of it. I was in and out of the hospital with few complications from the surgery.

If my emergency room visit had barely registered a blip on the radar, the same could be said for another health problem that I encountered in my twenties: Raynaud's phenomenon. It came on incrementally – so slowly, in fact, that I had plenty of time to make the mental adjustment to living the rest of my life with the same burdensome condition as my mother. Raynaud's, which constricts the blood vessels when the body experiences cold or stress, usually amounts to little more than a nuisance for the millions who suffer its numbing effects, which are generally limited to the fingers and toes. My mother had stoically put up with it her whole life. Why couldn't I?

જ

With only about 180 beds, St. Elizabeth's was a relatively small hospital, compared to some of the others in New York City at the time. I was assigned the four-to-midnight shift and quickly developed a nice rapport with my fellow nurses. Paychecks came every second Thursday, when we would often meet for lunch and a few laughs, the last of the big spenders.

After I had been there a year and earned a week's vacation, I elected to spend it working at Jewish Memorial Hospital, a city hospital in upper Manhattan that was looking for temporary help in the emergency room. The ER at Jewish Memorial made its counterpart in Dublin look tame. Police cars and ambulances streamed in one after another, and the parade of emergencies made for an overwhelming, eye-opening experience.

The weather was hot and muggy that week in July, and the hospital, which boasted air conditioning only in the ICU, felt like a sweatbox. Staff members, every one of us caked with dry perspiration, moved methodically from one emergency to the next, with no time to collect ourselves in between cases.

On my second evening there, a young Spanish-American man arrived with a bullet wound to the abdomen, and I was amazed at how tiny the bullet hole was as he was rushed inside on a stretcher. I had never seen a bullet wound before.

Seconds later, a woman suffering from a drug overdose was wheeled in. Her kidneys were failing and she was rushed from the ER to the ICU as soon as she was treated.

Each emergency room wasn't much more than a tiny cubicle. Between that and the hovering policemen and the stifling, still air, it was easy to feel oppressed by the conditions, claustrophobic even. So I was surprised to see a fellow nurse, a Filipino-American named Leda Chu, laughing as they whisked the woman away.

"What are you laughing at?" I asked Leda.

She smiled and asked, "Didn't you see her mother? She had two different shoes on."

"You clown," I responded. "You don't have time to look at someone's shoes."

It had already been an awful evening, but Leda had found a way to lighten the mood. I knew right away that I would like her, and indeed, we hit it off immediately. She took a job at St. Elizabeth's a short while later and often worked the night shift. Sometimes we did double shifts together. We quickly became friends, as did many of the other nurses with Leda. She lived in an apartment nearby, and several of us would often come by and chat after church on Sundays. If there was a wedding or something, she always did our nails; she was a wonderful manicurist. She had a knack for making us laugh as well, and her sense of joy was contagious.

Leda was also a practical joker. One night in the middle of a double shift, I was working the first floor and got a call from Leda, who was on the second floor, my normal floor. She told me she was missing three patients, and I naturally assumed she was joking. In fact, three young men, none of them seriously ill, had sneaked out for a drink. (It was Saturday night, after all.) When they returned from their night out on the town, their physicians duly discharged them.

Leda eventually married and had triplets, which left her ill and weak due to a blood clot that had traveled to her lungs. Her doctor advised her not to get pregnant again for a while, but she conceived a few months later. One cold morning she had to get a sonogram, and I picked her up to take her to the doctor's office. Despite having to drink several glasses of water and then hold her bladder, she was as bubbly as ever, smiling and telling jokes on the way to the hospital.

After she consulted with her doctor, she emerged from his office and said, "Maureen, it's four this time, not three."

I stared at her. "Please tell me you're joking."

She was. It was just one. But shortly after the baby was born, Leda discovered a lump in her breast and was diagnosed with cancer. Her health quickly deteriorated, and it became apparent that she wasn't going to survive.

I went to see her at the hospital one day and knew the moment had come. She was horribly restless and had been given an injection. Her husband was there, plus a few friends. As I stood by her bedside, it felt as if something was lifting me off the floor. I looked at Leda – she was so peaceful; she looked like an angel in bed – and then she stopped breathing and was gone.

I made many friends while working in health care, but none touched me the way Leda did. In the years to come, I would face my own mortality, and I would draw on Leda's glowing heart for strength. I still dream about her to this day.

ᘙᘊ

I remained in the health care profession for the better part of two decades. But as early as 1975, when I was working a swing shift at the hospital, I felt the urge to do something productive with my mornings.

After considering my options, I earned a real estate license and started working part-time as a rental agent for apartments. I welcomed the extra income, which I earmarked to help pay off my car loan. As for the real estate business, I viewed it as the perfect arena for me to exercise my competitive spirit – a quality I couldn't adequately explore in the nursing profession. Years later, when I gave up nursing and took on real estate full-time, I learned how radically different the two worlds really were.

By 1982, I had carved out a successful career as a nurse and had made a comfortable home for myself in an apartment in Hackensack, New Jersey. One of the tenants of my building, a single man who reeked of cigarettes, came by often to invite me to the parties he seemed to be constantly throwing. When he slipped a note under my door for an upcoming party, I decided to attend – a fortuitous decision, considering I met my future husband that Saturday night.

Bob Taylor, friendly and engaging, had recently lost his wife to a bone disease and had arrived at the party with another couple. He was forty-five and had begun to lose his hair in front, but he had a youthful face. Although not particularly athletic, he was slim and trim. He stood about my height of 5'8". We talked a while and he took my number, asking me if I would like to go out to dinner sometime, but I didn't hear from him for three or four weeks. When he finally called, he asked me out on a date – and I gladly accepted.

I liked him from the start. He was affectionate and clearly taken with me. But I could see from the beginning that he would want to get married. Although I felt comfortable when I was with him, I couldn't imagine myself marrying him. I resisted the notion, unwilling to rush into such a serious commitment. But as the days and weeks went by, I grew more and more fond of him until I suddenly realized I was in love with him.

We talked early on about his wife and her untimely death. The experience had left Bob bitter, especially toward doctors, for whom he had little respect or trust.

Bob didn't like dancing or playing sports like tennis or golf – three activities I enjoyed. He preferred instead taking a walk in the woods, or going for a hike. On weekends, we typically went out for dinner and then caught a Broadway show. We often stayed in New Jersey and attended a Broadway-type show, rather than make the trip into New York City.

We were wed in June of 1983. It was a lovely, intimate ceremony, attended only by a handful of close friends.

I moved in with him at his house in Wayne, New Jersey, and quickly found myself struggling with our new living situation. Along with the challenge of sharing a space with someone else, I found the extended commute to Manhattan close to unbearable. I was working a twelve-hour shift at the hospital. Combined with the commute, that made for a long day. After working with terminally ill patients all day, I came home exhausted to the core.

Finally I mentioned to Bob that I had a real estate license, one that I had barely used and hadn't renewed for years. What if I left nursing to become a fulltime real estate agent in New Jersey? The prospect of a short commute and a regular nine-to-five shift looked like a vacation. Bob was amenable, and I took the leap, saying good-bye to the hospital after fifteen years.

I had no idea at the time that, far from leaving my troubles behind, I had yet even to meet them. But I was about to.

❧ 3 ❧

The dream, though never quite the same, kept coming for me in my sleep, as if it had something to teach me.

I am walking toward the sea, where the waves rise and fall, ready to give chase. As I step closer, the path under my feet narrows until the water has closed in on me from both sides. The threat of drowning hangs over me like the leaden sky, and eventually I am forced to turn back, the waves continuing to pursue me as I scramble to safety. What would happen if I tripped and fell, if I gave in to the waves? I'm afraid to find out.

A husband. A new home and a new hometown. And now a new career. My life, after fifteen years of following the same arc, suddenly felt mysterious to me, like the waves that threatened to overtake me in my recurring dream.

I had landed a job with a local real estate company, but it hadn't taken long to realize that my personality – geared all those years toward nurturing and care-giving – didn't exactly jibe with the prototypical personality of a real estate agent. I had always had a strong work ethic, thanks no doubt to my upbringing on the farm, so I was prepared to tackle the challenge and succeed on my own terms.

But the first few weeks and months weren't easy.

My new boss, a successful businesswoman and my elder by several years, reminded me more than a little of my abusive schoolteacher back in Ireland, and I couldn't help but marvel at the fact that certain themes in my life seemed to disappear only to reemerge later.

But she was the least of my worries. The fickle nature of clients, the competitiveness of the industry, the salesmanship required both in person and over the phone – everything about real estate was a radical departure from the world of nursing. I missed my former profession and felt as though a part of my nature was not being expressed. I would eventually volunteer at a local hospice, politely turning down an offer to work full-time as a nurse while gaining what I needed: a chance to practice my nursing skills for a few hours each day. But for the moment, I concentrated on coming to terms with my new profession.

For the first several weeks, I began each day with the same morning ritual. I would savor a raisin bagel with cream cheese and sip a cup of coffee with milk on my way to work. Then, as soon as I had arrived at the office, I would volunteer to answer the incoming calls, knowing that I could claim any new clients who happened to dial our number. Thus I quickly learned my first lesson in real estate, which is that most prospective clients are just curious, not serious.

After being stood up, blown off, and taken for a ride for the umpteenth time, I decided a change in the routine was in order. Instead of going into the office and waiting for calls, I started to prospect door-to-door in my neighborhood, covering two or three blocks each day. Quite often I would be invited in for tea, and the next thing I knew I was fielding questions about Ireland from curious Americans who had never been to the mother country or had relatives on the other side of the Atlantic. I would finish the visit by handing them my card or a brochure from the office, inviting them to call me if they wanted to sell their home or invest in real estate or whatnot.

Over time, I slowly made the acquaintance of several neighbors, who ultimately became my clients. Thus the second lesson learned: people do business with people they know.

⌘

It probably wasn't practical, given my busy life, but by the time the holidays rolled around in 1984, I felt a strong desire to own a dog. Perhaps all those childhood attempts at hiding stray animals in my room back on the farm had finally caught up with me.

I had my hopes set on a golden retriever and talked incessantly about getting one to anyone who would listen. A coworker at the office only helped fuel the fire one day when she said, "I'll bet your husband gets you one for Christmas."

She didn't know Bob. An eminently practical man, Bob gave me a telephone for Christmas because ours had just broken. But by January, I had involved practically everybody at the office in my search for a faithful dog, and I soon learned about a West Highland at the pound: cute, little, white – the perfect prospective adoptee.

I called Bob at his office to discuss the possibility, and he replied warily, "Go ahead and look, but don't bring her home."

I delayed my visit to the pound by one day and used the evening to research the Westie breed, which I had never heard of before. My first step was to call my nephew Joe, who was somewhat of an expert on dogs, but what I learned from him – that Westies are awfully cute but typically bark a lot – was discouraging.

"Remind me to buy Joe a dinner to thank him," Bob quipped when I told him I was reconsidering whether or not to get the Westie.

Unfortunately for Bob, I made the cardinal sin of visiting the dog at the pound the next morning. Sickly, dirty, her coat a tangled mass of gray – she didn't look cute. More like wretched. And yet, somehow I felt drawn to her. As I stood there hesitating, my coworker Francine, who had come with me to the pound, laid on the guilt. "If you don't take her," she admonished me, "they'll put her to sleep, you know."

So I took the Westie – Bonnie – home, stopping on the way to the house to have her professionally groomed. After a bath and a shave, Bonnie looked like a bony little rat with runny eyes. As I studied her, I remembered a sickly cat I'd once rescued back at the farm.

When I got home, I called Bob at work to tell him about the new addition to our family. He accepted the news with a sense of humor, saying, "I hope you both have somewhere else to stay tonight." When he got home that night, he couldn't believe how pathetic Bonnie looked, a far cry from the noble golden retriever I'd first envisioned owning.

We noticed during our first few days with Bonnie that she *never* came when we called her. A visit to the veterinarian solved the mystery. She was deaf, thirteen years old, and would require plenty of tender loving care for the remainder of her life. The vet also informed us that Bonnie would need a hysterectomy, not to mention two teeth and a breast tumor extracted. She survived the multiple surgeries, helped along, no doubt, by the haute cuisine she enjoyed during her recovery. Having already turned her nose up at canned dog food, she bulked up on chicken and rice.

Six months later, Bonnie had gained weight, grown a fluffy white coat, and looked – dare I say – gorgeous. In fact, I think she knew as much. I caught her preening in front of the mirror one day and admiring her own reflection, as if she couldn't believe what she saw.

ᘓᘐ

The longer I stuck with real estate, the easier it got. I guess I shouldn't say *easy*. Though I was volunteering a few hours each morning at the local hospice, I still managed to log fourteen- and fifteen-hour days at my paying job. I spent countless hours on foot or in the car as I showed houses, checked in at the office, and made my rounds in the neighborhood.

But I was getting good at it, and I had the commission checks – suddenly rolling in now – to prove it. For someone willing to invest her time and energy, for someone willing to do whatever it took to be number one at her profession, there was a fortune to be made.

Of course, living life on the go *cost* me something, too. I had lost the one-on-one relationship unique to nurse and patient. That bond, built squarely on trust, was nowhere to be found in real estate. In its place: heartburn, anxiety, headaches, and insomnia.

Early on I noticed pain in my right shoulder – pain bad enough and persistent enough to send me to the doctor's office. It felt frozen, and I could barely move it. The doctor diagnosed it as bursitis, which sounded like a logical explanation to me.

But then one morning I woke up with a numb mouth, as if it had been shot full of Novocain. I had a cold at the time, and assumed it would go away. Instead, it became part of my morning routine. I greeted each new day confused and disoriented, caught in a strange, panic-stricken haze. I would drink a glass of orange juice, which helped quench my thirst and seemed to sharpen my ability to focus. But two hours later, after my raisin bagel and coffee, I could feel my whole body shaking.

It had to be the long hours. At least that was what I kept telling myself. Back home on the farm in Ireland, nobody had ever complained when they were in pain, and I wasn't ready to break from that tradition. Indeed, I knew that if anything, I should feel *grateful*. I had worked hard, and my hard work had enabled me to buy a dramatically higher standard of living than the one I had experienced growing up.

But strange aches and pains persisted. Soon they had spread to my feet and to my knees, to my *bones*, and the nurse in me couldn't help but register alarm. Were my symptoms tied to some form of malignancy? I had always been competitive, a go getter, maybe even a little hyper. Was I simply feeling stress? I coped as well as could be expected for someone still in denial. One bottle of Maalox and one bottle of extra-strength Tylenol: they rode shotgun with me wherever I went.

⊗⊗

Then came a particularly difficult set of clients. The husband, about 5'9", walked as though he had two left feet. The wife, a humorless homemaker, always wore a scarf, never smiled, and was absolutely vicious when she interrogated me or my coworkers. Both were in their fifties. Their twelve-year-old boy, meanwhile, acted more like their agent than their son. His habit of coming into the office while his parents waited in the car earned him the nickname of Little Jesus from my coworkers. "What do you have for us today?" he would ask.

I had already showed him and his parents dozens of houses. His grim mother spent forever in each house, after which she would walk out unceremoniously and offer no feedback. Though they were on a limited budget, they wanted the perfect house. Finally, after touring close to forty properties, they agreed on a three-bedroom split-level home, the seller of which was a woman in the midst of an ugly divorce.

Between the day the seller accepted our offer and the day we went to contract on the house, three months passed. During that time, my persnickety buyers made numerous inspections, each time finding something else wrong with the house – piddling little things they wanted the seller to fix. If the seller balked at making the repairs, the buyers demanded she reduce the price of the property. So back and forth they went, week after week.

Every Sunday the buyers made a pilgrimage to the house to make sure the seller hadn't done any new damage. Sometimes I was certain my clients expected the house to have collapsed into rubble in the seven days that had passed since their last visit. Not surprisingly, after a few weeks of this, the seller became increasingly infuriated, and what might have been a negotiation turned into an all-out, take-no-prisoners war.

Finally, after weeks of trivial and mean-spirited tit-for-tat, the two sides appeared ready to come to an agreement, so their respective attorneys set a closing date. My clients wanted to make a final inspection on the morning of the closing, so we set a time for an eight-o'clock walk-through.

When the day arrived, the seller called me at home and informed me that she had a problem. "The door to the bathroom," she explained. "You're going to have to stand in that doorway as your buyers go into the room because my ex-husband put his fist through the door and it's not fixed. I want you to stand in the doorway so they won't see the hole."

I was shocked and tried to dissuade her from such a foolish scheme, but she repeated her demand and then added another.

"I burned the countertop," she told me, "and I have a copy of *The New York Times* sitting on it. Just make sure they don't lift that newspaper!"

When I arrived at the house with the buyers, they barged inside and began inspecting the house before I had even removed the key from the front lock. The first thing they spotted was the hole in the skinny bathroom door, and it wasn't too long until they had discovered the huge round burn mark on the countertop under *The New York Times*. As they started to rant and rave about the new problems, I managed to shut them out long enough to think, *Oh, Lord! What a closing this is going to be!*

The closing lived up to its billing. The buyers and the seller fought even more dramatically than they had battled during the previous three months. And as they savaged each other, my head pulsed with an ache so severe my vision blurred. I prayed we'd be through by two o'clock, after which I would get myself some aspirin and a cup of tea.

But two o'clock came and went without a resolution, and I soon began to feel dizzy and nauseous. The argument had become a full-blown shouting match, with the seller jumping up in her chair and screaming across the table at my clients, and I could feel the blood pounding through my head. The two attorneys tried to calm their respective clients but couldn't, so they put them into separate rooms and proceeded to deliver messages back and forth between them.

We didn't finish until six o'clock that evening, by which time I was dreadfully sick: headache, nausea, dizziness. As had been the case with many other transactions at the time, I had no sense of my boundaries and had taken on the confusion of the clients. In fact, I often felt out of control, but I attributed my anxiety and the headaches and the sore joints and feet to the nature of the real estate business, not to mention all the other changes in my life. I had begun a new career in mid-life. I had married for the first time. And I was living in a new home and community. What did I expect?

Like others my age battling demanding work, I survived the tough spots with stimulants and painkillers. I downed my coffee everyday and swallowed plenty of aspirin. And I always carried my Marlboros with me.

No one could have convinced me to slow down.

ᗇᘐ 4 ᗇᘐ

At the same time I started working at the real estate agency, another newcomer arrived at the office: Donna Powell. A tall redhead with an unforgettable laugh, Donna boasted a playful sense of humor and a delightful presence. With her freckles and turned-up nose and a head full of curls, she was downright sprightly.

One night while out on a listing appointment, we met with an Italian-American couple. The husband was the boss of the house, a classic and domineering patriarch. The wife, meanwhile, played the submissive role, sitting in a chair with a basket in her lap and folding grape leaves, never saying a word. While the man of the house rambled on about selling points and whatnot, the wife simply nodded her head in agreement.

On the way out, I asked Donna what she thought of their relationship, and she responded lightheartedly, "Oh, they're just airheads." It was the first time I had heard that expression, but it wouldn't be the last time that my colloquial vocabulary grew thanks to a turn of phrase from Donna.

But she was more than just my mentor. As the days and weeks flew by at the office, Donna became my confidante. If I needed advice or just an ear to chew, she was always there for me. Growing up on the farm, I had learned to keep my feelings to myself, but I was slowly shaking that poor habit loose.

When my health continued to deteriorate, I shared my symptoms with Donna, who offered an off-the-cuff diagnosis. "I think you could be having bouts with low blood sugar," she surmised one day at the office. "You should see a doctor."

I took her advice, and one visit to a local doctor confirmed Donna's theory: I was diagnosed with severe hypoglycemia, as well as allergies. The cure? Cut out stimulants from my diet. Coffee, refined sugar – even my trusty Marlboros were given the heave-ho, which was no small task. Not surprisingly, the cloud of depression that had been threatening to overtake me receded, and physically I began to feel noticeably better. But not for long.

Though I had addressed the doctor's concerns, I soon developed numerous aches and pains and frequently felt a burning sensation in my esophagus, which traveled to my shoulders before climbing into the left side of my head.

To soothe the migrating pain, I still kept an oversized bottle of Maalox with me in the car as I drove from appointment to appointment. A constant passenger, it sat between the two front seats. When the pain was too much, I would unscrew the cap, throw my head back, and choke down a dose. The relief was usually immediate, but ephemeral. Two hours later, the heartburn would return in full force. When it did, I accomplished whatever mental gymnastics were necessary to explain away the symptoms. "Well," I would tell myself, "I fell off the wagon and had a cup of coffee today," or, "I shouldn't have had that fast food for lunch. Of course I have heartburn." I knew my lifestyle was contributing to the heartburn, but I tried to convince myself that as long as I had my trusty bottle of Maalox with me I'd be all right.

When rationalizing my symptoms away didn't work, my training as a nurse kicked in. "Maybe I have an ulcer," I worried one day. "Maybe a heavy cream diet will help." I started to eat more cream, but it didn't do much good. I still finished every meal with a Maalox chaser.

ᘒᘒ

By October of 1986, an uncomfortable rash, itchy and persistent, had appeared on my hands and my feet. Creams, topical ointments – nothing made even a dent in the prickly, creeping sensation. I finally found temporary relief by immersing my hands and arms in hot water up to my elbows. But the problem, too severe to ignore, sent me to a general practitioner.

Tall and rail-thin, Dr. Peabody was a soft-spoken, almost taciturn man. When he looked at my hands, he seemed truly baffled.

"Well," he said quietly, "I don't know what's causing the swelling." He suggested that I might be pre-menopausal and prescribed for me Lassix, a diuretic.

I was skeptical of his guesswork. Pre-menopause, as far as I knew, was not associated with so much swelling or such a persistent rash, so I asked Dr. Peabody if he thought the symptoms might indicate a more serious condition.

"No," he responded, "I don't think it's serious. But let's do some blood work to see what we can find out."

I filled the prescription for the diuretic, which made me urinate frequently but did not bring down the swelling. When my blood work came back from the lab, most of the indicators looked normal, but the sedimentation rate, which indicates inflammation, was unusually high at thirty-four millimeters. The typical rate for a healthy female is zero to twenty.

Dr. Peabody, though, didn't seem concerned, and I slowly began to grasp what he couldn't: that perhaps I was in trouble. Worse still, I couldn't help feeling like he wasn't *that* interested in finding out exactly what was wrong with me. In fact, it felt like he was more interested in simply writing me a prescription and sending me home.

My shoulder pain, meanwhile, still plagued me. I had been visiting a chiropractor, a handsome young man who would arrive at his office each morning in a hefty pickup truck. But like Dr. Peabody, he seemed to be groping in the dark. I would describe the pain to him, and he would do an adjustment in my spine or my shoulder, or he would try hot packs or ice or even one of his machines. Nothing helped. Sometimes his efforts seemed only to accentuate the pain.

When winter rolled around, the itchiness finally disappeared, but other symptoms worsened while new problems surfaced. My feet had turned purple and had swollen so much that I could barely bend my toes. Perhaps not surprisingly, the soles of my feet hurt when I walked. My hands and fingers, too, had turned a sort of brownish-purple, and they throbbed constantly. Simply bending them elicited pain.

In February, by which time I had begun to gain weight, I made another appointment with Dr. Peabody. Still unalarmed by my symptoms, he offered a new diagnosis: arthritis. Instead of pressing him further – or going in search of a second opinion – I accepted his pronouncement that I was entering pre-menopause and was suffering from mild arthritis. By downplaying my symptoms, Dr. Peabody had given me what I wanted: the green light to keep running hard while denying the warning signals from my body.

But my body, not accustomed to dealing in half-truths or head-in-the-sand denial, would find a way to be heard.

❧ 5 ❧

Something was coming for me. It seems obvious now. But at the time I couldn't name it. I couldn't see it. I could hardly feel it. The mysterious disease, a steamroller incapable of mercy, was bearing down on me steadily, incrementally, wanting only to flatten me. But I remained blissfully in denial about the slow and steady decline of my health.

As it had in the past, it would use a traumatic event, in this case the death of my beloved Westie, to lumber ever closer. Bonnie, the pathetic fur-ball turned loveable old dame, had become an indispensable member of our family. She was playful, affectionate, and loyal to the end – and she eventually helped pave the way for two more Westies in the family: McDuff and Kerry. But in March of 1987, a little more than two years after I had first brought her home and Bob had grudgingly accepted her, Bonnie succumbed to congestive heart failure. Her death left me numb with grief.

Two years earlier, it had been the difficult clients. The episode had triggered in my health a precipitous decline. Now, two days after losing Bonnie and crying my heart out, I felt physically battered by my anguish. The numbness in my face that I had experienced periodically as a child while trying to fall asleep had returned in full force, stripping away any feeling from my nose and my upper lip, as if I had been given multiple injections of Novocain. In addition to the numbness, I felt a burning sensation in my eyes and in my forehead, plus a throbbing pain in my jaw. The combination was enough to make me feel like an alien in my own skin. My face felt so numb and so strange that I couldn't help feeling horribly uneasy. Did I have a brain tumor? Cancer?

Instead of consulting a doctor, I waited fearfully for the symptoms to disappear. When I came down with a cold a few days later, I felt relieved. Clearly the pressure from the oncoming cold had caused the strange sensations in my face and head.

But a week later, nothing had changed. I finally realized it was time to visit a general practitioner who, upon listening to me describe my symptoms, recommended I see a dentist.

The dentist assured me there was nothing wrong with my mouth, certainly nothing that could be causing the numbness and pain I was experiencing.

Perplexed and still worried as I drove home, I decided to simply live with the symptoms and hope that they would go away.

☙❦

I missed Bonnie. She was irreplaceable. Yet I suspected, as did Bob, that finding a new dog would at least partially fill the emptiness I felt in her absence. Bob and I discussed the possibilities and agreed that perhaps two dogs would be better than one: they could keep each other company. So I set about finding another Westie – or two.

I didn't have much luck until I learned of an elderly breeder on a farm in Connecticut who was about to put up eighteen Westies for adoption at the humane society. I called Bob about the opportunity, and he quipped, "Oh, my God! You're going to come back with all eighteen in the car!"

He suggested I adopt a female, but when I arrived at the humane society all the females had already been spoken for. Only one Westie remained: a big male. He looked awful and sat in a cement cage with no bed. I asked the attendant to let him out so I could gauge how he behaved.

As soon as he was loose, he leapt into my arms and put his paws around my shoulders. I couldn't let him go. It was as if he were begging me, "Please, take me with you." His nose was dry and he was in rough shape, but I gave a donation, signed the papers, and off I went with my new canine companion: McDuff.

Bob was standing in the front yard when we got home, and McDuff gave him the same treatment, jumping into his arms as soon as he was out of the car.

McDuff smelled terrible, so I took him straight to the bath and scrubbed him clean. As soon as I had blown him dry, he got comfortable on the couch, making himself at home. He seemed perfectly content until that night, when I left him in the kitchen in a nice little bed I had made for him. I closed the dog gate and went upstairs, and as soon as I lay down he started bawling.

"I think you brought home a handful," Bob groused.

I went down to comfort McDuff, but he started crying again the moment I left. This went on for a while until I finally found some old beach towels in the basement and warmed them up in the dryer. I put one on McDuff's bed and the other over him after he lay down. From that night until his death years later, he never cried again. But he always had to be covered at night.

A few months later I would pick up Kerry, a Westie puppy and the perfect playmate for McDuff. But for now, we pampered the adorable new addition to our family. I missed Bonnie, but I had found someone just as special in McDuff.

∽∾

Though my mom had always come after my stray cats and dogs with a broom, my father had always had a soft spot for them. He had, in fact, a special relationship with animals, one built on tenderness and respect. Thus it seemed a bitter twist of fate that he fell ill with a severely enlarged prostate a few weeks after Bonnie died.

When I flew to Ireland to see my dying father, my symptoms for the first time became more than just troubling; they became a nuisance. My hands had swelled to twice their normal size, and my feet and legs, along with being swollen, felt cumbersome and hard. The visit, already emotionally painful, was exhausting physically as well. But I told no one of my symptoms. My brothers and sisters and I had been taught not to complain, and old lessons died hard.

As for my father, it was apparent to all of us, including him, that death was near. He had been receiving care from a visiting nurse when I arrived, but my siblings and I wanted to get him to a hospital for better, round-the-clock help. My mother seemed divided about how best to proceed: on the one hand, she didn't want to put him in a hospital; but on the other hand, she didn't want him dying at home, either.

So I finally confronted the two of them together one day and said, "Dad, where do you want to be?"

"In my own house," he answered.

"Then that's where you're going to be," I said.

But Mother protested, saying if she were in his place, she would not want to be a burden to anybody.

I was furious with her. This was my father's home, where he had been born, where he had worked and toiled his whole life. Because of her own fears, she couldn't allow him the last wish of dying in his own home.

As I reflected on the dynamics between them, I realized my father was equally to blame: he too often gave in to her unreasonable demands. Though she appeared to be the weak person, she ultimately ruled the roost.

We took Dad to a hospital in Dublin, and Mother stayed home. She didn't feel comfortable traveling. At the hospital, my father and I spent several hours reminiscing.

"You know, Maureen," he said during one visit, "I'm ninety years old. I never felt old until I reached ninety. You must remember this is old machinery."

I didn't want to hear that. My father had always been young at heart, with a quick mind and a generous spirit. He had ridden a bicycle until his mid-eighties, when his knees finally protested. But *he* was not a complainer. He lived life to the fullest. He had always seemed so in tune with every aspect of his life: his family, his animals. Most of all, he loved the land. He sensed its beauty, the divinity behind it. He had no formal education but had worked hard all his life. He was a strict Catholic.

Finally I answered him in a joking tone. "Maybe you need to find a new body. Then you'd be able to come back."

"Maybe sometime," he said quietly.

As with many of the conversations with my father during my visit, it was hard not to feel overwhelmed by emotion. I often had tears in my eyes. I knew that death was near for my father, and I couldn't help wondering if these were my last days as well.

The morning I was scheduled to fly home, I stopped by the hospital for one last visit with my father, and we talked about my childhood.

"Are you still gathering up cats and dogs?" he asked.

"No," I said. "You know Bob would never allow me to have more than two dogs."

Dad then recalled something that had happened when I was ten years old. I had found a sick cat under a tree alongside the road and brought it home. I had been carrying a basketful of groceries and had placed the cat right on top of the unwrapped groceries. When my mother saw that, she hollered at me to take the cat back where I had found it. It was cold – the middle of November – and the cat was weak (pregnant, too, as I would later find out), and I didn't feel right about returning it to its roadside home.

My mother insisted, though, and continued hollering at me until Dad came up the driveway and asked what all the hullabaloo was about. When I told him, he lobbied for a compromise: I could keep the cat for the night in a banana basket in the barn.

The episode remains etched in my memory. My father, as tender as he was strong-willed, knew me well and shared the same love for animals. When he spoke, he spoke honestly. He spoke from the heart. Whenever he could, he tried to make the world a softer place for those around him.

As I said my final goodbyes, I knew I wouldn't get back to Dublin again to see him. My body, too, was failing, and I knew it. I left for Shannon Airport in near agony. Unable to take the pain any longer, I stopped on the way to the airport to find a pair of shoes that were large enough to accommodate my swollen feet. I normally wore a women's size 8, but I barely managed to squeeze my throbbing feet into a men's size 11 sneakers.

After my visit to the shoe store, I found a drug store that sold Dr. Scholl's foot wraps, and as soon as I arrived at the airport, I hurried to the restroom and wrapped my feet. The men's sneakers, the wraps – neither helped much, but I was desperate for relief and had a long plane ride ahead of me. If nothing else, the wraps alleviated the pain I felt in the soles of my feet as I walked.

Back home, I had barely parked my car in the garage when I resolved to seek out an endocrinologist immediately. Several of my symptoms – the puffy eyes, swollen feet, and weight gain – indicated to me that I might have a thyroid problem.

I found a doctor in Midland Park, New Jersey, who was young and highly efficient – probably the most capable person I had come across so far in my quest for answers. She sat and listened patiently as I recounted my symptoms. She then ordered blood tests and called a couple days later with her assessment.

"Your thyroid functions look normal," she said, "but you have elevated antinuclear antibody levels at 1/380. This may indicate a problem with connective tissue, so you need to see a rheumatologist."

She had been unable to connect the dots, but she had narrowed the scope of the problem.

My husband, though, was indifferent to the news. Since my first visit to the doctor, he had seemed annoyed, sometimes even reacting with sarcasm as I tried to fill him in on what I had – or hadn't – learned after the latest trip to the doctor's office. The diagnoses had run the gamut from hypoglycemia to allergies, from a problem with my teeth to a connective tissue disorder. But none of the doctors I had consulted had managed to pinpoint precisely what was wrong with me. Nor had any been able to alleviate any of my symptoms.

As my health plummeted and the source of its drop remained a mystery, Bob grew silent and intractable. I understood his frustration. I, too, was near the end of my rope. But I couldn't understand his lack of support. Why was he blaming *me*?

In retrospect, it seems clear that he didn't think there was anything truly wrong with me. He could have joined in my quest for answers, but to him the whole thing looked like a wild goose chase – one concocted in my head, no less. He didn't go with me to my appointments, didn't offer any sympathy, didn't do anything to assuage my fears. During those awkward moments when I tried to involve him in my struggle, he seemed dismissive of the problem. He didn't want to hear about it.

"Can't you see my face is changing?" I would ask, desperate for someone to take me and my failing health seriously.

He would shake his head and respond, "I don't see anything wrong with you."

I was alone.

❧

It was a hot summer day when I arrived at the rheumatologist's office for my 11 a.m. appointment. I had a two o'clock closing that afternoon in Hackensack and hoped to be done with my appointment and back in town for lunch before the closing. With that in mind, I showed up a half hour early, determined to give myself ample time for the visit and any tests that might be administered. But it wasn't until 11:30 that the nurse finally ushered me into an examination room and handed me a paper gown to slip on.

As I sat shivering in the air-conditioned examination room, I battled another attack of Raynaud's phenomenon. I had been living with the bothersome condition for several years now, but lately the attacks had become more frequent and more debilitating.

I could hear the rheumatologist wandering the corridor on the other side of the door, talking to his staff and whatnot. What was taking him so long?

An hour later, my hands and feet had turned purple. I was still waiting, still shivering in my thin paper gown, still wondering where the hell the rheumatologist was. At this rate, I was going to miss lunch – and maybe even miss my closing appointment.

I could see and hear the wall clock ticking off each second, and when it reached 12:30, I finally lost my patience. I opened the door, glanced down the hallway, and spotted a nurse. "Look," I said after flagging her down, "I've been sitting in this room since eleven-thirty and my appointment was for eleven o'clock. Where is the doctor?"

"Oh," she responded, "he's had an emergency."

Apparently, she didn't realize I'd heard him walking up and down the corridor for the last hour. I knew he had overbooked his appointments – a common practice among doctors.

"I have five more minutes," I said firmly. "I have to get out of here because I'm a real estate agent and I have a closing at two. So either he comes in to see me or I leave."

That was all it took. A few minutes later, the doctor entered holding my chart. He was a tall man whose arrogance was palpable. Without looking at my hands or feet or any part of me – and without apologizing for keeping me waiting for two hours – he announced in an authoritative voice, "You have lupus. I'm going to write you a prescription for plaquanil."

"Whoa," I objected, "wait a minute! What is wrong with my face? I have a numb face."

"Well," he said with a shrug, "that's Sjogren's Syndrome."

"No," I protested once more. "It can't be. I don't have dry eyes, and I don't have a dry mouth."

He seemed surprised to hear me challenge him. "What do you know about dry eyes and a dry mouth?"

"I'm a nurse," I answered.

"Well, what are you doing selling real estate?"

The question was an accusation as much as it was an inquiry, and the next thing I knew we were trading insults.

Finally he said, "You know, I don't like real estate agents. I had my house listed with one who was such a dingbat that I had to sell the place myself."

"Well," I said, no longer caring if I offended him, "I guess you feel the same way about real estate agents as I do about doctors like you."

That was the end of my appointment. I left in a hurry for Hackensack, but not before paying $250 for the privilege of waiting two hours for five minutes of the good doctor's time.

∾ 6 ∾

The old adage about boiling a frog is based on a simple though, in some ways, counterintuitive truth: an immediate threat is far less dangerous than an incremental one. If a frog is dropped into a pot of boiling water, it instinctively leaps to safety. But if it is placed into a pot of lukewarm water and only slowly brought to a boil, it won't know the difference until it's too late.

I guess I was fortunate to see that I was in trouble, that I had to do *something* – and soon – lest my slowly disintegrating health fail me altogether. But I felt like the heroine in a bad horror movie. I was the only one who recognized the peril I faced. Everyone around me – the doctors and experts and even my own husband – thought I was nuts.

My visit to the arrogant and condescending rheumatologist had been a bust, and I didn't bother filling the recommended prescription for plaquanil. His bedside manner – not to mention his hasty diagnosis – had left me cold.

I had read about an endocrinologist in Baltimore named Dr. Saul Nielson who I thought might be able to help me, but the soonest I could get an appointment to see him was in August, several weeks away.

So it was back to my family physician in Wayne. By now it was clear he found my complaints irritating. I suppose he thought I was a hypochondriac, mentally unstable, or both. I didn't help my case when I asked for a referral to see a neurologist. It seemed wise to me to get a brain scan in order to rule out the possibility of a brain tumor or growth that might be causing the numbness in my face. My doctor only reluctantly agreed.

The neurologist he referred me to, meanwhile, was a cold, detached man. After battling an acute bout of claustrophobia during the lengthy brain scan, I arrived at his office to learn the results. He was sitting behind his desk and had a severe expression on his face. I braced myself for the worst.

"Mrs. Taylor," he said soberly, "the results from your MRI are negative. I strongly suggest that you seek psychological counseling."

I was floored. To a degree, he was right. I *did* need counseling. But not because I was a hyperventilating hypochondriac with nothing better to do than chase after a phantom diagnosis. I needed counseling because I was battling a terrifying unknown – alone. And now those entrusted with my care were beginning to question my grip on reality.

"Do you realize how sick I am?" I asked in disbelief.

He dismissed the question, in effect dismissing me and whatever it was that was stalking me.

I wanted to throttle him. I wanted to grab him by the collar and shout, "Look at my hands and feet! They're swollen! Even my face is swollen!" But I kept my thoughts to myself. Rather than waste energy on someone so heartless, I was determined to find a doctor who would take me and my illness seriously.

☙❧

On July 31 at three in the morning, I awoke to the phone ringing. I had been expecting the call and wasn't surprised when I picked up the receiver and learned the news: my father had finally passed away.

A few hours later, I got out of bed and found a stray cat I'd never seen before loitering by my front door. It rubbed up against my legs, and I couldn't help sensing my father's spirit. It was as if he had sent the cat to wish me a proper farewell. My neighbor Joan eventually adopted the stray cat, who I would often look after while Joan vacationed in Florida.

As for my father, I knew he was finally resting in peace.

❦

A published author and an expert in his field, Dr. Saul Nielson had all the credentials of a highly regarded endocrinologist. Thus, when my August appointment rolled around and I finally met him, I was surprised to find him a wonderfully down-to-earth man. He was warm, spoke candidly and informally, and seemed to me to meet the profile of the ideal doctor, the type of doctor someone in need of care could readily trust.

The drive to his office had taken three hours, but I immediately felt welcomed by his courteous staff, all of whom seemed genuinely concerned about my welfare. Finally, I had found help.

I handed him all my medical records, including the results from the test that showed my antinuclear antibody count at 1/380 with a speckled pattern. I didn't understand at the time what the results indicated; only later would I learn that the ANA count could predict the severity of several diseases classified as autoimmune.

As soon as Dr. Nielson had reviewed my records, he ordered more tests. When they came back, he was able to confirm that I did not have lupus. Instead, he thought I might have a connective tissue disorder of unknown etiology. Regardless, he thought my biggest problem was allergies, so he ordered several skin tests to isolate the allergens that were causing the negative reactions in my body.

I returned to Dr. Nielson's office every three months for the better part of a year, and during one of my visits he prescribed for me a thyroid hormone. It seemed to help a little, but I continued to experience pain, swelling, and hardness in my feet and legs. Worse still, I was beginning to have difficulty walking and using my hands. On my bad days, simply turning the key in the ignition felt like a full day's work.

I felt a sense of creeping desperation. I hoped and prayed Dr. Nielson would be able to find an explanation for my symptoms, but at the same time I could sense already that no simple treatment would cure whatever it was that ailed me. Something was very wrong.

☙❧

As my symptoms continued to deteriorate, I tried to keep the developments to myself. I didn't want to burden anyone with my problems. And the person who should have been my biggest supporter – Bob – remained resentful toward me and my illness.

I was still making an effort to get to the office each day, and because of that I think Bob assumed that my health problems, if they existed at all, were relatively minor and certainly manageable. He refused to discuss my illness with me, and he still denied the existence of my body's slow disfigurement. He saw no swelling in my face, feet, or hands, claiming he saw nothing different about them or me. I still prepared dinner for him each night, and we still ate together, but an ever-widening gulf stood between us. He never asked about my trips to Baltimore, much less accompanied me on the three-hour journeys. And I no longer pressed him for support.

In retrospect, I know it was fear that drove his behavior. He had already lost his first wife to a terminal illness. The idea of losing me was clearly too much to bear. So he shut down, denying my illness and distancing himself from me emotionally. His was self-protection at any cost – even if that cost meant losing the very person he feared losing. Self-inflicted loss was a more attractive alternative, I guess, than admitting he had no control over the future.

☙❧

That winter, my health took another sharp downturn. Raynaud's phenomenon – that cumbersome and frustrating condition inherited from my mother – continued to plague me, only now more often and more severely. My body felt weak, and I had difficulty with the simplest of tasks, such as lifting my hands over my head. My abdomen had become distended, and when I tapped it, it felt like a tightly tuned snare drum. I was retaining fluids; thus despite my efforts to remain hydrated, my urine output was scant.

I began to wonder if I had an abdominal tumor. It was another shot in the dark, but I was groping for any clear-cut diagnosis now, and I think I actually found comfort in the idea that I might have a tumor. Tumors could be identified and treated. They could be shrunken, removed. Yes, they could cause death. But at least I would know the cause of my decline. It seemed patently unfair – not to mention mystifying – that after all the tests I had undergone, I still had no clue what was chasing me.

When I began having difficulty opening my mouth, Dr. Nielson sent me to a reputable but expensive dentist in Baltimore, and the dentist diagnosed me with TMJ, or Temporomandibular Joint Disorder, a relatively common problem with the joints that connect the lower jaw to the skull and one that can cause everything from jaw pain to headaches. It seemed a logical explanation, but the mouth guard the dentist fitted me with only made the pain worse. I used it only briefly before giving up on it. I could hardly open my mouth by now.

Finally, by the spring of 1988, my condition had become so severe that I could no longer endure the three-hour trip to Baltimore for my checkups with Dr. Nielson. I was crushed to lose contact with him after a year under his care, but something had to change. Dr. Nielson and his team had given me hope, treating me with respect and dignity while trying to find the cause of my illness, but I wasn't getting any better. I was getting worse.

The first dehumanizing aspect of my illness presented itself in July, when I finally realized I could no longer chew my food. I adopted a liquid diet – soups, puddings, and so on – and began liquefying all my meals, putting everything I could into a blender.

The racket and the mess drove Bob crazy. "Why can't you chew?" he would ask irritably.

I didn't know. *Nobody* knew. My whole face and head had grown numb. My sense of taste had gone, and I had difficulty getting food into my mouth. My swollen hands and feet were in a constant state of pain. My skin felt like leather – hard like Formica. And nobody could tell me what was wrong with me.

7

So often in life there exists an irreconcilable difference between what we want and what we need. What do we call that divide? What name do we give to the space between ego and wisdom, to the way we somehow stumble upon our own salvation? Kismet? Serendipity? Dumb luck?

With my health steadily crumbling and my body feeling less and less like my own, what I wanted more than anything was relief, quick and complete. I wanted to know what was hounding me, I wanted the magic pill that would make it go away forever, and I wanted my old life back. A stressful but lucrative job, a comfortable marriage, a predictable routine – everything that I had taken for granted before suddenly felt like the height of happiness.

But what I *needed* was power. *Courage*. I needed to meet my illness, to stare it in the face, and to show it the door. I would need help from others, but ultimately my health would be my own responsibility. To be accountable, I would need to change everything about myself: what I ate and drank, how I breathed and moved, what I thought and believed, what I wanted from life.

The seeds of my metamorphosis came in the form of a little book, given to me by Eileen Amrian, a friend and fellow churchgoer who was suffering from similar, though less severe, symptoms. The book, written by Dr. McPherson Brown and already three decades old at the time, was called *The Road Back*, a fitting title for the role it would play in my own healing.

In it, Dr. Brown claimed that people could recover from rheumatoid arthritis, lupus, and a disease I'd never heard of before – scleroderma – by taking an antibiotic called tetracycline for an extended period of time. Dr. Brown had built up a successful track record with the antibiotic, administering it to his patients and achieving the hallmark of success: full remission.

As I read the book, I began to see myself – my inexplicable symptoms, my failing health – in some of the patients Dr. Brown described, and I felt a tiny surge of optimism when I learned that Dr. Brown had started a clinic in Virginia. I couldn't possibly travel that far for treatment, at least not on my own (I was having difficulties dressing myself by now), but I called the clinic nonetheless, hoping they could point me in the direction of someone nearby who subscribed to Dr. Brown's theories and would prescribe his antibiotic therapy.

I was given the name of a rheumatologist in New Jersey – Dr. Hal Whitman – and I quickly phoned for an appointment. But Dr. Whitman's earliest opening wasn't until several weeks away, in late August.

I could have waited it out, but I knew I needed help now. I gave the book to a doctor who was married to a friend of mine. After reading it, he agreed that Dr. Brown's theories held promise, so he wrote me out a prescription for tetracycline.

At first it seemed to make a difference, but by late July, I had progressed from being mildly disabled to grossly disabled. I felt bowled over by weakness and was experiencing shortness of breath, and my whole body felt cold. I had lost all feeling in my head and face, and I had lost my sense of taste. Once again, it felt as if I had been given a mammoth shot of Novocain. I was numb from forehead to chin, inside and out. On top of that, I felt a strange burning sensation inside my nose and right eye.

One day after struggling my way through a short walk in the neighborhood, I returned home and was shocked to find a dead fly in my eye. Had I not bothered to look in the bathroom mirror, I wouldn't have even noticed it – because I certainly couldn't feel it.

A wave of utter dread overtook me. *What* was *wrong* with me? I began to wonder if I was already dead and just didn't know it yet. Fear gave way to doubt. Was it all in my head? Did I really need psychological help? I suddenly felt old. *Enfeebled.* Something like this, I told myself, could only happen to someone running out of time.

Other symptoms steered me toward the same conclusion. I could hardly swallow anymore and was beginning to feel undernourished because I could only eat what I could liquefy. Mealtimes had become an exercise in humiliation. Because I no longer had any feeling in my mouth or lips, I slurped and gagged on my food, just as one would do after a visit to the dentist's office, often drooling and coughing as I ate. I was forced to wear a bib and to clean up after myself as one would an infant.

Bob, meanwhile, continued to live in an almost comical level of denial. How he could think I was the same vivacious woman he had married five years earlier was beyond me. But he stubbornly remained unsupportive, refusing to take my illness seriously.

I couldn't help but respond with an anger bordering on rage, and I found myself wishing my symptoms on him. If he could spend an hour in my body – just one hour – he would know what it felt like to be me: the numbness, the burning, the humiliation. But he was incapable of empathy. Had his first wife's death drained him of that virtue?

⊙⊙

I can't say precisely when I knew I was dying, but sometime during July of 1988, the realization crystallized. Every step had become a monumental effort. Simple tasks exhausted what little strength I could muster. My hands had begun to curl inward, and I could no longer flex my fingers. My arms, meanwhile, felt like they had been fastened to my body. If I tried to extend them or lift them above my head, the skin on my chest, already stretched tight, would send shockwaves of pain through my body. My skin had begun to resemble a wild animal's hide – or the surface of a conga drum: parched, tough, and discolored. It had receded around my mouth, exposing my teeth.

The tetracycline hadn't worked. My body was failing, and thus far nobody in the medical profession had been able to help me. I was beginning to wonder if there was a road back.

⊙⊙

By the time I arrived on August 28 for my appointment with Dr. Whitman, my feet were hard and swollen and had ballooned in size. My legs felt like dead weight, and it was all I could do to lift them. I could barely walk and found stairs next to impassable. My hair had begun to fall out, and even though the hot August sun was beating down on me and roasting the pavement beneath my feet, I felt it necessary to don a woolen cap and winter gloves as I hobbled from the car to Dr. Whitman's office.

The thought returned: maybe I'm dead and I don't really know it. *Maybe I'm just walking around in somebody's dead body.*

Eileen, my patient chauffeur, waited in her compact Honda. I took one last glance back at her and then paused in the middle of the parking lot to take off my hat and gloves so that I could smooth my hair. Maybe indulging my vanity made me feel more connected to the living. Regardless, I knew deep down it was a futile effort. Nothing could have made me look anything other than grossly disfigured. My face had become as distorted as my feet.

I entered Dr. Whitman's tiny office and was escorted by a nurse to the examination room. I knew nothing about Dr. Whitman, but I knew he represented my last hope. When he appeared in the doorway of the examination room, I was immediately impressed by his imposing 6'5" figure.

He entered without greeting me, his hands stuffed into the pockets of his white coat. He stared at me for what seemed like an eternity, and I felt as if the sick me – the *dying* me – was being seen for the very first time.

Finally he spoke, not to me but to the illness. "How long have you been like this?"

As I answered, he took my hands in his, then pinched the skin on my face, all the while looking through me at the disease. It wasn't so much an examination as it was a calling out. He knew my face. Knew my deformity. Knew my pain.

"You have scleroderma," he told me, and my mind raced as he shone the spotlight on my pursuer, finally identifying what the others had been unable to detect. He defined it, explained its causes and side-effects, and answered each of my questions with precision and patience.

I had scleroderma. Systemic sclerosis. An autoimmune disease. My body was producing too much collagen. My body's connective tissue – in my skin, my lungs, even my heart – was hardening.

His words echoed in my mind. "We don't know what causes it, and we don't know how to cure it. It's progressive."

I showed Dr. Whitman all of my medical records to date, including a fairly recent one that showed my ANA test result: a dilution of 1/5,550 with a speckled pattern.

"That's extremely high," he said. "Almost off the charts. I want to do some tests today. Some blood tests. And I'd like you to have a pulmonary function test. After we do those, I can get you onto some kind of treatment protocol."

The mention of tests snapped me out of my fog. "I'll do the blood tests," I said, "but I don't have the energy to huff and puff through another pulmonary function test. You'll just have to use the results from the test Dr. Nielson gave me. It's in my file. I think it shows that my lung capacity's dropped to around forty-two percent."

"What other symptoms are you experiencing?" Dr. Whitman asked. "And what treatments have you tried?"

I told him that I could barely chew or swallow and that I was liquefying all of my food. I also told him that I had heard about the renegade antibiotic treatment for rheumatic disorders that Dr. McPherson Brown had advocated and that I was taking tetracycline.

"If I had seen you before you started the antibiotic," Dr. Whitman said, "I would have prescribed a different drug. Tetracycline can be too fiery for the system, particularly for a patient already in the inflammatory stage of scleroderma."

It was hard not to feel optimistic. Finally, *finally*, I had found someone who could name my illness and – better than that – talk knowledgeably about it.

Before I left his office, I stirred up the courage to ask for a prognosis.

"Well," Dr. Whitman answered, "your disease is advanced, but we have some drugs that can slow it down."

I have never experienced anything comparable to the loneliness, the despair, or the fear I felt at that moment. My mind raced. *My God*, I thought, *my body is broken. I can't sleep. I can't enjoy the smallest pleasure, like eating my raisin bagel on the way to work in the morning. I feel so . . . uncivilized.*

The thought of living what was left of my life in a body made of stone was too much to bear. Would I end up in a wheelchair? A nursing home? I had nowhere to go. No one to turn to. I felt utterly alone.

I was afraid to die.

୭୧ 8 ୭୧

While a nurse working with the sick and dying, I had learned a fundamental truth about my patients: the terminally ill often know their fate before their doctors do. Sometimes a patient would tell me she knew she was dying. And sometimes I could see it in her eyes that she already knew the truth. Either way, the doctor was usually the last one to know.

So it was in my case. As I said goodbye to Dr. Whitman and his small staff and stepped outside into the hundred-degree heat, I felt a strange sense of relief. I had known for weeks that I was dying. Now it was official. Moreover, now I knew what was killing me.

I tugged at my wool cap, pulling it snuggly over my ears. Eileen was still waiting for me in her tiny Honda, and I was thankful for her support. But at the moment I wanted nothing more than to be alone. With my pursuit of a diagnosis finally over, I needed time to think, time to digest. Knowing something in my heart was different than having Dr. Whitman spell it out for me in clinical terms.

I was dying. *I was dying.*

I stooped over and tried to cram myself into the passenger seat, huffing and puffing as I struggled. The numbness, the swelling, all the pesky symptoms were still there, but I was overwhelmed by the sheer exhaustion I felt. I tried to tell Eileen the news, but no words came out. Finally, after some prodding from her, I managed to share what I had learned in Dr. Whitman's office.

"At least you have a diagnosis," she replied optimistically.

I barely heard her. I was still absorbed in my own thoughts. My body felt foreign to me, almost as if it was my enemy, and I wondered how long I could possibly live in it. How had it deteriorated so completely without a diagnosis until now? How was it that all the time and resources I had spent chasing a diagnosis had, until today, amounted to nothing? How could there be nothing – no treatment – for this disease?

As we drove home, Eileen suggested we stop for lunch.

"No," I protested numbly. "I feel cold as ice."

"Then let's go get a bowl of soup somewhere," she insisted. "It will warm you up."

I tried to object and once again found myself explaining that I couldn't eat solid food, that I had to liquefy everything I ate, that even then I made a degrading mess of myself. But Eileen was insistent.

I finally relented, and we stopped at a restaurant. As soon as we stepped inside, I regretted the decision. The air conditioning was cranking chilly air, and sure enough, I found myself in the grip of a brutal Raynaud's attack. I ordered the cream of broccoli soup, but when it arrived at our table I was trembling so badly that I could barely lift the spoon to my mouth, which, in turn, was so numb I couldn't tell whether the soup was hot or cold. For all I knew, the soup was scalding my lips and mouth and my throat on the way down. I wanted to forget the world – the world I was leaving. I wanted to curl up and die.

I felt annoyed with Eileen, meanwhile, because she didn't seem to comprehend the weight of the news I'd been given. She told me to have faith in God, which seemed ludicrous at the time. I didn't think much of a God who could deal me such a blow.

Finally we left the restaurant, and Eileen drove me the rest of the way home. When I got inside, I collapsed in a heap on a chair in the living room, where I sat for an hour, numb with grief, devoid of energy, and overpowered by fatigue. I felt utterly weak.

Bob came home from work a few hours later and mumbled a hello. He knew I'd been to see a new doctor that day, but he didn't bother to ask about my appointment. He was withdrawn, and as usual his presence only succeeded in accentuating his absence. He was there in body only.

As I blended my dinner, he prepared his own. My thoughts drifted to happier times when we had enjoyed dining at cozy restaurants together. Those days were gone.

When we were finally seated at the table, Bob asked, "Well, what did the doctor say to you today?"

"He told me I have scleroderma," I answered.

"Well," Bob snapped, "how long will it take you to get better?"

I gazed at him and said without blinking, "There is no cure. It's progressive."

Bob looked at me incredulously. For a moment, he appeared flummoxed. But after a brief pause he threw down his knife and fork and walked away from the kitchen table.

So much, I thought, *for "in sickness and in health."* I tried to put myself in his shoes and wondered how I would have acted had the roles been reversed. It was difficult to do because the present moment overflowed with so much tension.

Bob never spoke another word to me that evening. I wanted to kill him.

☙❦

The following Friday evening, four days after my appointment with Dr. Whitman, I felt an acute sense of dread as I lay down to sleep. A deep chill ran through me, and I shivered. Every movement – however small – seemed a great labor. It had taken everything I had to put on my night clothes. As I tried to get comfortable, I felt too much pain on my right side, so I switched sides and then piled up several pillows to support my body.

I finally drifted off, but I slept fitfully and only partially, dozing for fifteen or twenty minutes at a time. Around midnight I awoke to the sound of someone moaning, and suddenly I realized the groans were coming from my mouth. I was feverish and disoriented.

As I shivered in the dark, I felt wave after wave of splintering pain shooting through my shoulders, my knees, my spine. Would the pain kill me before the disease? I knew I needed relief – some aspirin – but I felt so weak I could barely push myself up into a sitting position before getting out of bed.

As I made my way down the stairs, I leaned hard on the railing, stopping every few steps to sit down and rest and to get my bearings. I could hardly see the stairs – or anything else that required a downward gaze – and my skin felt ready to snap, it was stretched so tightly around my eyes.

By the time I got to the kitchen, my hands and feet were blue from another Raynaud's attack, and I was shaking uncontrollably. I fumbled with a bottle of baby aspirin and mixed several of the tiny pills with water. Later I guessed the total at twenty. Not one went down easily. I choked and gagged and forced each one down, undeterred by the number of tries required. I knew instinctively that I needed to get some fluids into my body, so I coughed down as much water afterward as I could.

Then it was back upstairs, the struggle floating by in a timeless fog. I stumbled to the guestroom, determined not to disturb Bob, and propped myself up on as many pillows as I could find. As I lay down, my heart beat so hard it felt like a bass drum exploding in my chest. The pounding was so violent and so profound it felt like it was coming not from within me but from outside my body.

I'm going now, I thought. *I'm leaving my body.*

Gradually my heartbeat slowed, the pounding replaced by a distant pulsing, and my brain waged war on itself. "Go ahead," one side said. "You should die. You have nothing left." The other tried to pull me free from the darkness. "Stay. Don't go. You have reason to live." Back and forth they fought, two voices vying for a commitment from me.

As I held court with myself, the argument slowly morphed into an unlikely lullaby, and I eventually surrendered to sleep, content to wait for an uncertain future.

ᎶᎧ

I woke up alive on Saturday morning. The aspirin had worked. The fever was down.

As soon as I could, I pulled myself up out of the guest bed and called Dr. Whitman's office, where I left a message with his answering service. I suddenly felt lucky for having discovered Dr. Whitman at what felt like the final hour. Finally I had found a doctor I trusted.

But when the return call came from the answering service, Dr. Whitman wasn't on the other end of the line. The voice, so kind and reassuring, belonged to a gastroenterologist named Dr. Gibbon. After I told him about my symptoms – and what I had been through the night before – he reacted with genuine concern.

"You need steroids," he said. "I'm putting you on prednisone. A pretty high dose: eighty milligrams." Then he asked, "Do you know anyone who can give you an injection of depo-medrol, or can anyone drive you to an emergency room for one?"

I told him I knew a nurse – a friend of mine named Marilyn – who would give me the injection, so he said he would call in the prescriptions to my drugstore.

Before hanging up the phone he added, "I'm very concerned that you're having such a hard time swallowing. You need nourishment. If you don't improve within the next few days, you may need hospitalization."

The thought of checking into a hospital – the tests, the x-rays, everyone poking and prodding at my body, possibly being fitted with a gastroenterology tube – petrified me. I didn't know if I could survive the depersonalization of a hospital experience, especially given how degrading my condition had already become.

After I hung up the phone, I asked Bob to pick up the prescriptions from the drugstore. He agreed to go, but only after I insinuated that Marilyn could do it if he wouldn't. As little as he wanted to do with me or my illness, he still had his pride. I doubt he wanted others to think poorly of him.

Still, he told me he had to finish up some yard work first, and it was two long hours – during which time I drifted in and out of sleep – before he returned home from the drugstore with my prescriptions.

I felt like I had endured an eternity by the time he handed me the small white bag. I immediately took a dose of the prednisone and then got on the phone to call Marilyn; I still needed her help with the injection.

Bob, meanwhile, went back to his yard work. He stayed out all day without ever coming back inside to check on me. I suppose I shouldn't have been surprised by his response, given how he had reacted to the news earlier that week, but it seemed unfathomable to me. Instead of feeling sad or even angry about my prognosis, he acted as if he was simply annoyed. He was as aloof and as remote as a perfect stranger, which was what he was becoming to me.

In hindsight, I often wonder if the prednisone sent him over the edge. Prednisone – a powerful drug with potentially serious side-effects – had helped hasten his first wife's disease, ballooning her weight in her final weeks.

But as Bob tended to his garden that day, I felt utterly abandoned. I was lucky to have a close-knit group of friends at the office, as well as others, such as Eileen and Marilyn, who were eager to help me out whenever they could. But in my own home, I was alone. The man who should have been my closest confidante and most devoted care-giver had already been down this road once – and refused to travel it a second time with me.

❧ 9 ❧

By evening I began to feel a little better, and by the time Monday rolled around, I felt almost human. My skin was still hard and tight, but I felt stronger. The swelling in my face had gone down a little, and I was experiencing less pain.

I called Dr. Whitman's office first thing that morning to make an appointment and landed one for the following day.

I was eager to learn more about what I was up against, and Dr. Whitman supplied me with more information when I arrived for my appointment. "Your blood tests are back," he said after greeting me. "You have what we call a mixed connective tissue disease with overriding systemic sclerosis. The blood test results also indicate that you have anemia and a slight elevation of urea nitrogen and creatin. Your lungs are affected. We've got to get you on some kind of protocol right away."

Part of that protocol was to cut my prednisone dose in half, to 40mg, which Dr. Whitman prescribed in 5mg pills so I would always be conscious of how much I was taking.

Dr. Whitman then informed me that I would need to collect my urine for the next twenty-four hours so it could be analyzed. He would be keeping me on the Armour thyroid that I had started taking when I was still in Dr. Solomon's care, plus adding several other medications to my regimen, including D-penicillamine, minicycline, and procardia.

The D-penicillamine made me nauseous, so I stopped taking it after one day. My use of minicycline was equally short-lived; it gave me a rash. So Dr. Whitman set me up with doxicycline, a milder antibiotic, instead. As for the procardia, which was supposed to improve my circulation, it made me weak, so Dr. Whitman substituted cardizan. But it, too, didn't agree with me, so I ended up not taking anything for my circulation. Months later I would learn that taking fresh garlic – cut up into tiny pills for easy swallowing – could help on that front.

I hadn't wanted to take drugs, much less a veritable potpourri of them, because I knew some of them, such as the prednisone, were a package deal that included the potential for severely toxic side-effects. But I also knew I couldn't live from day to day without medication. In fact, I probably would have taken any drug Dr. Whitman prescribed – without question – if I had thought it could relieve my pain. And the prednisone *did* make a significant difference: it decreased the pain, alleviated my debilitating weakness, and gave me strength to go on.

But the drugs did more than give me relief. They pointed to the possibility, however remote, of recovery. No drug illustrated this more than the doxicycline, which Dr. Whitman prescribed in three-day cycles. I would take 100mg each day for three days, then wait three days before taking the antibiotic again.

When I finished the first three days on the drug, I thought I noticed some newfound flexibility in my hands. But after taking the prescribed three-day hiatus, my hands swelled again. After another three days on the antibiotic, I noticed more flexibility – just a little – but the stiffness returned once again during the waiting period. The pattern continued for weeks. Each time I took the drug for three days, I saw slight improvements. And each time I went off the drug for three days, my health deteriorated, and I seemed to slip backward. The fact that the antibiotics were clearly having an impact on the symptoms gave me confidence in Dr. Brown's theories in *The Road Back*.

After a month on the doxicycline and with October coming to a close, I realized I wanted to know more about Dr. Brown's antibiotic therapy, so I decided to call him in Virginia one evening. A lady with his answering service fielded my call, and when I asked if there was any possibility of talking with Dr. Brown himself, I was astonished to be rewarded with his home phone number. I stirred up the courage to call him at his home, where a woman answered.

"May I speak with Dr. Brown?" I asked politely.

"Certainly," the woman said. "May I ask who's calling?"

I told her my name and admitted that I'd never met the doctor before but that I was seeing someone his office had recommended and that I was hoping to learn more about his antibiotic theory. She seemed satisfied with my response, and I felt a surge of excitement as the doctor and author came to the phone.

Dr. Brown spoke in a fatherly voice, like a wise and kind old professor, and I found myself pouring my heart out to him. I told him about my symptoms – how short of breath I was when I walked, how tired I was, how numb my head and face had become – and I let him know that I had started antibiotic therapy and was eager to learn whatever he could teach me about his theories.

"Who's your doctor?" he asked in his gentlemanly voice.

"Dr. Hal Whitman," I answered.

"You have nothing to worry about," he said. "You've got the best and the brightest." He went on to reassure me that I was on the right track. The fact that I was taking prednisone, he told me, was a good thing indeed. In his estimation, I wouldn't be able to withstand the side-effects of the antibiotic treatment without it. "I think you'll be okay," he added in an encouraging tone.

The best and the brightest. I hung up the phone feeling guardedly optimistic. I had two doctors – both of them well qualified and caring individuals – in my corner. One had inspired me to search for answers. The other would, in the months to come, help guide me out of the abyss.

Is there anything more healing than the human touch? All the drugs in the world couldn't have given me what Diane Latteiri, a physiotherapist and family friend who lived in the area, bestowed upon me when we got together for our morning sessions at my home. Thanks to a prescription from Dr. Whitman, my new regimen included regular visits from Diane.

Young and pretty, with beautiful dark hair and the quintessential Irish complexion, Diane was the product of an Italian father and an Irish mother. She was highly qualified – both as a physiotherapist and as an emotional healer. She plied her trade elegantly, teaching me how to move and slowly loosening the tissue around my face and the fascia around my head. From our very first session, she immediately and intuitively tuned into my illness, employing her gentle art to open up my joints and increase my circulation. She became in a short time the equivalent of my confidante, often listening to me as I unloosed in therapeutic monologues the crippling fear I was battling.

After a few weeks of seeing her, I began to sense a difference in how I moved, how I felt. My joints were opening up, and I could sense an increase in my circulation.

But Bob questioned the usefulness of the therapy. All he could see in Diane's regular visits was another claim to be made against his company's health care plan. Would he lose his health insurance because of me? Would he lose his job?

I didn't – and still don't – think his fears were rational, but soon his worries degenerated into an ultimatum. If I wanted any support from him, he informed me one fall evening, I had to give up my physical therapy.

The dilemma cast a spotlight on the helplessness I often felt within my marriage. Instead of making do on my own, as I had for all the years I'd been single, I was suddenly dependent upon someone else for my health care, my healing now a hostage to Bob – and his fear.

"Do you understand what Diane is doing for me?" I asked, feeling myself ready to boil over with frustration and resentment.

"It's only a massage," Bob responded.

"No," I snapped, "it's actual physical therapy."

"Then go out and take a walk," he countered. "That will move your limbs."

By now I was hardly able to get into the office on a regular basis, much less exercise. But Bob's denial knew no bounds. I had a terminal illness, and he was worried about keeping his premium health care benefits. In time, I would take charge of my own healing. But for the moment I was trapped. I had no choice but to cancel the sessions.

ᏬᏋ

One night that fall a powerful storm blew into New Jersey, and as luck would have it, Bob was out of town and I was alone in the house. Sort of. As I tried to drift off to sleep, the wind rattled the house, and McDuff banged on the kitchen gate downstairs.

I went to him and tried to calm him, but he wasn't having any of it. Finally, I brought him and Kerry upstairs to the bedroom with me. Bob forbade the dogs from coming upstairs, but . . . well, what he didn't know wouldn't kill him.

I picked up McDuff and put him on Bob's pillow, and McDuff, having finally had his needs met, turned his back to me, rested his head on the pillow, and promptly fell asleep. Kerry, meanwhile, got comfortable on the floor, and I laughed at the thought of how Bob would react to the dogs' new sleeping arrangements. Fortunately, he didn't come home early from his trip.

❦ 10 ❦

We don't know what causes it, and we don't know how to cure it. It's progressive.

Since my first visit to Dr. Whitman, part of me had tried to deny the scope of my illness. I wanted to believe that I was going to beat the disease, even if no one else before me had reversed its deformities. Yet Dr. Whitman's honest but bleak assessment hung over me, a constant reminder of what lay ahead. The remainder of my life, for all I knew, might be measured in months. Or weeks.

And what kind of life would it be? Weak. Disfigured. Drooling on myself as I choked on my liquefied diet. Doped up on a whole menu of powerful meds. If scleroderma didn't kill me, the cure would.

Dr. Whitman, whom Dr. Brown had championed as the best and the brightest, had identified the disease stalking me. But the most that Western medicine could offer me was a slow, medicated death. Scleroderma was a progressive illness. There was no turning back. No such thing as a full remission.

I guess it shouldn't have come as a surprise then when I, a former nurse schooled in traditional Western medicine, slowly opened myself to other methods. Desperation had trumped training. Intuition – sometimes blind, sometimes illogical – now counted as much as knowledge, maybe more.

I would still need conventional medicine; Dr. Whitman's support and knowledge would be crucial. But just because others had drawn a line in the sand between traditional and alternative medicine didn't mean I had to; I could benefit from both sides.

In November, I entertained an intriguing suggestion from Donna at the office. The sprightly redhead with the infectious laugh and an abundance of can-do optimism thought it was time to experiment with a new approach.

"You should try a macrobiotic diet," she offered one day.

"Macrobiotic?" I asked. I knew nothing of the subject.

"It balances the yin and yang energies," Donna explained. "When the body is balanced, it heals itself."

Yin and yang? Balance? I was ready to try anything. I took my closest friend up on her offer and had her make an appointment for me with a macrobiotic counselor on the other side of the state.

Two nights before my appointment, I had a vivid dream that I was attending a funeral for the NBC news reporter Martin Fletcher. The funeral home was actually a restaurant, and I walked inside carrying two huge suitcases that were weighing me down. I lowered the suitcases to the floor, one in each hand, and then looked up to take in the dining area and its blue-and-white checkered tablecloths.

The next morning I woke up and tried to decipher the dream. What did it all mean? I knew Martin Fletcher hadn't died; I'd just seen him on the news the other day. The suitcases seemed symbolic. Was I ready to unload some baggage?

I rode with Donna the next day to the Sojourn Inn, a restaurant used by the macrobiotic counselor and his clients. I was flabbergasted to see that the restaurant bore a striking resemblance to the one in my dream from two nights before, right down to the blue-and-white checkered tablecloths. We sat down to a macrobiotic supper, and afterward the woman who hosted the meal, a wonderful macrobiotic cook, told us about her husband Fletcher, who was dying of cancer but was too stubborn to adhere to the diet she had prescribed for him.

We then went upstairs to a little office and met with the macro-biotic counselor, who was a dead ringer for the news reporter Martin Fletcher! He had the same voice and the same thin face.

I was stunned by all the similarities to my dream but sat down to learn as much as I could about the macrobiotic diet. The diet, he explained, included grains, vegetables, and several sea vegetables with names I'd never heard of before. The list of prohibited items was extensive and included milk, wheat, yeast, meat, sugar, and caffeine. I would get my protein from beans, tofu, and wheat gluten.

He then began to explain the etymology and history behind the diet. Macro meant *complete*, and the diet was designed by a Japanese man named Misu Kuichi. The success of the diet, he pointed out, depended on its intricate preparation, which included specific ways of cutting – and chewing – the food. "You need to chew each bite fifty times," he said.

As I listened, I realized I would have to modify the program if I wanted to follow it at all. My hands had become like claws and were barely functional, and it had been months since I'd been able to chew solid food. How would I prepare and eat the food correctly? I con-fessed that I liquefied my meals.

"That just won't do," he informed me. "You'll lose the energy inherent in the diet if you put the foods in a blender. It won't work."

Though he'd been a macrobiotic counselor for years, he had never heard of scleroderma. He designed for me instead a diet tailored toward cancer patients. He also recommended that I place hot ginger packs on my kidneys as part of my new regimen.

I left the meeting knowing I would have to customize everything about the diet. How would I prepare the food, much less chew it? I would stick with the blender. How would I apply the ginger packs when Bob refused to have anything to do with me or my illness? I would have to find a way.

I began following the macrobiotic diet religiously the very next day – after going grocery shopping with Donna. For breakfast, I blended miso soup, tofu, brown rice, and greens with warm water left over from steaming vegetables. For lunch, I blended the steamed vegetables with beans and rice.

Then there were the sea vegetables; the memory of my first encounter with them makes me laugh to this day. At the time, I had lost all sense of taste, which turned out to be a blessing in disguise because I could still *smell* the sea vegetables – and they smelled awful. I've since acquired a taste for them.

I continued to cough and choke as I drank my blended macrobiotic meals, and I still wore a bib to catch whatever dribbled down my chin. I looked like an infant learning how to eat for the first time and was too mortified to eat in front of anyone.

Except for Bob. I'm sure he didn't like what he saw, but we continued to share the dinner table, usually sitting across from each other in silence as we ate. I don't remember him ever asking me how I felt during those meals. Even at his level of denial, he must have noticed my deterioration. But he maintained a stoic silence, unable or unwilling to inquire about my health. I suppose he felt frightened, but I don't think he knew how to express his fear without withdrawing.

I wanted to help him, but I had just enough energy to meet the demands of my failing body. I knew to survive I would have to pour everything I had into the healing process, physically, emotionally, and spiritually.

As for the ginger packs, I drummed up the courage to ask Bob for his help, but he refused, wanting nothing to do with the unorthodox treatment. So, necessity being the mother of invention, I found a way to administer the ginger packs – on the toilet. The ginger packs had to be warm and had to be changed often, and sometimes my hands were too stiff to wring out the cotton, but I persevered with my little pot of ginger. I would place the warm packs against the back of the toilet seat and press my kidneys against them for a short spell, each interval bringing palpable relief to my kidneys while fortifying my resolve to heal myself.

After a few weeks on the macrobiotic diet, I began to notice positive results. The food calmed my digestion, and the practice uplifted my spirits. For the first time since falling ill, I had become an active agent in my healing. I was engaged in a planned, positive, and prescribed practice designed to help me get well.

I called the macrobiotic counselor twice after our initial meeting to talk about the effects of the diet and to make adjustments, but each time I called, I felt let down. Instead of recognizing my limitations and helping me to adjust, he kept urging me to abandon the blender, insisting I cut and chew the foods according to strict macrobiotic principles. He urged me to make another appointment each time I called, but I didn't see the sense in traveling so far to see a practitioner who couldn't tailor his advice to me or my condition.

In what would become a recurring theme of my recovery, I continued with the diet, but only after modifying it to work for me. I didn't always combine just the right ingredients, and I didn't cut up the vegetables in the precise manner prescribed by the principles of the diet. Sometimes my carrots went into the pot whole for cooking. Sometimes they even went into the pot with the tops on. Despite the little heresies I committed each day, the diet seemed to be balanced enough, giving my digestive system a much-needed rest.

After several weeks on the macrobiotic diet, I realized I needed more instruction from an expert, so I called the Macrobiotic Institute in Boston to see if I could find the name of another macrobiotic counselor closer to home.

The institute referred me to Elaine Nussbaum, a macrobiotic counselor based in West Orange who had written a book on her own healing from cancer. When I called her, she told me that in addition to counseling she also taught cooking classes. I wasn't well-versed in macrobiotics, I told her, but I'd been on the diet for a month and it seemed to give me a sense of peace.

At my first meeting with Elaine, she listened attentively to me while offering up encouragement. When I told her that I needed to liquefy my food, she responded, "If that's the way you have to eat, then that's the way you have to eat. You're getting really good food. You're not following macrobiotic principles one hundred percent, but at least you're getting good nourishment."

Elaine charged a hefty hourly fee for each appointment, but I felt the price was worth it and visited her again several times. After each appointment, I came home feeling supported, encouraged, and sometimes even optimistic.

ᏜᏬ 11 ᏜᏬ

One step forward. Two steps back. Much to my chagrin, I was finding that the road back didn't follow a straight line, that it was possible to gain momentum one day only to lose twice as much ground the next. I was slowly learning to fight for every inch of progress. But some days were worse than others. Some days, everything looked bleak.

Although I felt somewhat revitalized by the macrobiotic diet and was faithfully taking the medication Dr. Whitman had prescribed for me, neither gave me what I really wanted, which was hope – rock-solid and undeniable. The macrobiotic diet made me feel appreciably better, but its healing properties were slow-moving and at times inscrutable. The drugs, meanwhile, merely managed the symptoms of my disease. They could not prevent further deterioration.

As fall gave way to winter, I found it harder and harder to press on. My skin – still drawn tight – pulled at my features and continued to distort my face. My right eyelid sagged, and my mouth contorted as I spoke, drawing to one side each time I moved my jaw. Talking, in fact, had become a tiring ordeal. My jaw felt as if it had been clamped shut, and my tongue felt like a lifeless wad in my mouth, independent of my control. The numb-yet-burning sensation in my face and head had intensified, as if a radical neurological transformation was under way inside my skull.

During each appointment with Dr. Whitman, I would inevitably ask what was foremost on my mind: would my face ever look normal again? Would I ever regain normal use of my claw-like hands? And each time Dr. Whitman artfully dodged the question, telling me he had never seen a reversal of the deformities caused by scleroderma.

On Christmas Day, four months after my diagnosis, Bob and I traveled to my brother's house, where we ate the traditional holiday feast with Chris and his wife. As I struggled to eat my mashed potatoes – the only item on the menu I could chew – no one said a word about my clearly declining health, other than to tell me I looked emaciated.

But a few days later one of my relatives dealt a blow to my all-but-lost self-esteem when he casually mentioned during a phone call, "I can't believe how much you've come to look like your Uncle James."

The comment was painful and hurtful – but enlightening. Now I understood my family's reticence to acknowledge my suffering. Uncle James, whose strange legacy still haunted us all these years later, had battled his crippling health problems for years before finally passing away, his body contorted by a disease no one understood. I could still see his gnarled hands, which mine had come to resemble so much, and I could still see him frowning grimly at the dinner table as he struggled to wield a spoon. After my grandfather had died, Uncle James had lived out the rest of his life alone on the farm, at peace with his disease and his deformity but a mystery to us all.

To this day, I often wonder how he managed to get by as long as he did. But then I invariably remember one of our family's favorite stories about Uncle James – the sort of story that puts his resilience into perfect perspective.

When I was growing up, the priests would stand before the congregation once a month during Mass and read aloud the "dues," which usually amounted to a couple of shillings that each person or family that lived in the parish was asked to pay to the Church. People who hadn't paid up were made an example of at Mass, their names trotted out for all to hear. It was a cruel custom, especially in a poor rural area where the Church often overvalued someone's land or possessions and demanded more of them than they could actually pay.

Such was the case with Uncle James, who worked alone on his farm without the aid of children or a spouse yet was expected to fork over a sizeable sum to the Church every three months. It was hard enough for him on cold winter mornings even to get to Mass. I can still see him struggling down the road on his bicycle on a frosty winter morning. He had somehow managed to learn how to ride a bicycle despite his deformity.

Uncle James always came to our house for Sunday dinner, and one Sunday he arrived in a foul mood, having learned that the Church, after studying the value of his land, was requesting he contribute more. He sat down, furious, and began railing against the Church.

"They should give *me* money instead of asking me for money!" he growled.

Mother, supremely superstitious and fearful of doing anything to offend the priests, protested. "James," she said, "please stop talking bad like that about the priests because everything you say about them they can read in their prayers in the morning."

Uncle James looked at her askance and said, "They can read it in their ass! I could care less!"

❦

Like most sufferers of scleroderma, I was learning that the pain and the discomfort amounted to only half of the disease. The other half – strange and unsightly disfigurement – left me a stranger in my own body. Though the prednisone had helped bring my swelling down, my mouth and lips looked even more shrunken than before, leaving my teeth fully exposed. The skin on my face pulled so tightly that I couldn't smile, and it hurt to talk. Each time I looked in the mirror, I was shocked to see a deformed face staring back at me. It was alien. Somebody or something else. Not me.

I reached the nadir of my disfigurement when I realized I no longer wanted to be seen in public. The naked truth, though a bitter pill to swallow, was that I wasn't the only one horrified by my deteriorating appearance. My face shocked strangers, as well as those who hadn't seen me for some time.

As the scleroderma forced my body to produce more and more collagen and my skin drew ever tighter, my face and body took on the hallmarks of the disease: my lips had all but disappeared, my mouth hung open, and my purple hands and fingers looked more like claws, gnarled and perpetually curled inward. Sometimes while driving I would glance at the contorted and ulcerated hands gripping the steering wheel and gasp, "Lord! Those can't be mine!"

But I couldn't remain hidden forever, and one day while making a trip to the grocery store, I spied a woman whose house I had sold a few years earlier. I glanced away, wishing in vain I could disappear, but she spotted me and asked as she frowned and squinted at me, "Is that you, Maureen?" From the look on her face, I could tell what she was thinking: *My God! What happened? Did some hack mess up a facelift?* I told her I had been ill, but I didn't have the courage – or the energy – to go into the details.

It hurt to know that my appearance shocked people who hadn't seen me in a while. Had I fallen ill with cancer instead, or some other life-threatening internal disease, I could have more readily explained to others what was wrong with me. And my explanation would have likely met with a compassionate shake of the head or an empathetic frown. But scleroderma wasn't exactly a household name.

Of course, in our culture, appearances – especially for women – are just shy of everything. Youth, vitality, beauty – billions of dollars are spent each year in the commercial sector to corner the market on immortality. I was not immune to those pressures.

Nor was I impervious to my upbringing. My mother had reminded me countless times that I was an unattractive child, and now scleroderma hammered the point home. When I looked at my disfigured face in the mirror, I recalled my mother's habit of pointing at unattractive people and then whispering in my ear, "You look just like her" or "He's almost as ugly as you."

She mercilessly went after my nose, which was turned up slightly at the end, and I remember standing in front of the mirror as a kid and pulling it down, imagining what it might look like without the tiny lift at its tip.

Scleroderma answered that question. The skin on my face, taut and hard, had pulled my nose down, erasing what I had only recently come to accept as a lovely distinction. I remembered the comments of the plastic surgeon, that I had a nose countless of his patients would have paid anything to possess. And I remembered the pettiness and the meanness of my mother, who seemed intent on cutting me down as a child. Slim, 5'8", and with a pale complexion and sparkling blue eyes, I was, in fact, an attractive woman, and I had realized as much after escaping my mother's destructive clutches to carve out a life in the States.

But scleroderma, like my mother before it, had cut me down to size, playing on my insecurities and stealing my self esteem.

"When you admire yourself in the mirror," my mother had told us more than once while we were growing up, "the devil's looking over your shoulder."

✂ 12 ✂

As 1988 drew to a close, the prospect of dying continued to haunt me. I had closed the books on a tumultuous, frightening year. Would the new one be my last?

Occasionally a friend would stop by and momentarily lighten the mood, but I spent most of my days feeling despondent, whiling away the hours in the den, where I sat gloomily on a loveseat by the window. I would let my mind float in and out of consciousness, following it wherever it led. I had nowhere to go but inward.

I contemplated practicing meditation – something I had flirted with more than a decade earlier after taking a Sylva Mind Control course in Paramus, New Jersey. But the visualization and relaxation techniques I had learned fourteen years earlier looked quaint now – and impossible.

I felt desolate, totally consumed by my misery. My declining appearance, my estrangement with Bob, my utter loneliness – everything conspired to make my prognosis seem that much heavier, that much more certain. I was dying, and nothing could change that.

Finally one afternoon while sitting in the loveseat and dredging the depths of my grief, I heard a still, quiet voice. *You always were,* the voice said as the evening sun flowed in from the west-facing window, *and you always will be.*

The voice belonged to my past, to a strange, dream-like experience one morning long ago, when I had been a nurse and had still been living in New York City. My alarm had coaxed me out of a deep sleep into a semi-dream state on that hazy morning, and in the half-light between waking consciousness and the subconscious world I had heard a voice speak the same words: *You always were, and you always will be.* The voice had come to me in a dream, but it had sounded so real I had been tempted to glance around the room in search of its owner as I had climbed out of bed, and as I had walked the corridors at the hospital that day, I had turned the phrase over and over in my mind. *What did it mean?*

Until now I had forgotten the incident. But here was the voice again. *You always were, and you always will be.* The voice, calm and full of certainty, seemed to be prompting me forward, encouraging me to face the future without fear.

But part of me wanted only to die. I felt I had nothing left. I had lost my health, my husband's love – even my ability to work. I still forced myself to get up each day and dress for work – often with the help of my neighbor Sandy, who would help me with my buttons or a zipper on those days I dared wear something more complicated than a pullover. And I still stopped in at the office each day, but I could barely manage the energy for a twenty-minute visit. Beyond that tiny commitment, I preferred to hide from my family, friends, and coworkers, avoiding their phone calls and retreating into myself.

Yet the mysterious phrase continued to echo in my ears. If part of me was ready to die, the other part – the part willing to listen to the voice – was ready to heal.

☼

Healing meant taking responsibility for my future. It meant letting go of my pain – or at least finding the courage to move forward in spite of it. On my good days, when I still had hope, still had energy, I resolved to make my healing the primary focus of my life. I already knew the worst-case scenario. What did I have to lose?

I continued working with Elaine, whose influence extended well beyond her macrobiotic teachings. I learned from her that garlic could help with circulation and even boost the immune system. The practice was simple: take a clove of garlic, cut it into pill-sized pieces, and swallow them with water. It wasn't long before my circulation began to improve. In the months and years to come, I would use garlic to fight colds and flu as well.

Elaine also encouraged me to walk a little bit each day, telling me that I needed to find a way to get some exercise. She motivated me to get moving, but when I started walking in January I could only take a few steps before I would have to come back inside and sit down. I felt frozen to the bone whenever I went outside, and the bitter cold made me feel nauseous. But I knew that even a tiny bit of exercise would help my body while halting my deteriorating coordination. So I kept trying. Some mornings I would barely set foot outside before having to turn around and return home, but each morning I made myself go back out again and take at least as many steps as I'd taken the day before.

Quite often, the walks were frightening, even disorienting. I would feel lightheaded, as if I was about to faint, and I would lose my concentration. Where was I? How had I gotten here? The cold cut through me, and while I couldn't do much about my feet and hands, which were already purple with Raynaud's phenomenon, I could protect my face. I bought a ski mask that covered everything but my eyes, mouth, and nose. I never went far from home. And I always planned my routes so that, if I had to sit down in a hurry, there was a park bench or something to rest on nearby.

My cardiovascular system, I learned during one of my appointments with Dr. Whitman, simply didn't have the capacity to support me on my walks. The same was true of my renal system, which couldn't receive blood fast enough. Thus the almost surreal lapses of concentration, the unsettling disorientation.

But I pressed on. Long enough, in fact, to have other, equally troubling experiences.

ᘒᘓ

I often longed for a deep sleep, for death, and one frosty January morning while dragging my body into my car and feeling like a seal trying to maneuver on dry land, I contemplated suicide. The thought flashed through my mind: it would be so easy simply to close the garage door and let the engine run until the fumes filled my lungs. I didn't want to part with my life, but I desperately wanted out of my body and all the pain attached to it.

What I didn't know at that moment was that I had already reached rock bottom. Plenty of dark days still awaited me. But the spark of my recovery – the will to change and to learn – had already caught fire. I just couldn't see it for the darkness. In fact, although there would be several turning points for me in the coming months, January was already turning out to be a watershed month in my recovery.

At an appointment that month with Dr. Whitman, I unloaded a few demons, telling him that I wanted out of my body, that it wasn't working.

"Depression comes with the territory," he said. Then he made me squirm, asking, "What kind of support are you getting at home?"

"None," I admitted.

Dr. Whitman nodded knowingly. "When it comes to supporting a spouse suffering from a serious illness," he said, "husbands usually fall into two camps: they either disappear or totally take charge of your care."

"Well," I said, "he hasn't disappeared yet, but he hasn't done too much, either." I left it at that, declining to tell him how truly angry at Bob I had become. In fact, I no longer gave a damn what he did or said because he was no longer the man I thought I had married. I sometimes prayed that he would be touched by illness in order to be made more human, but he got stronger on my prayers.

Dr. Whitman urged me to see a psychiatrist, which I did that very day, eventually finding a psychologist for regular counseling. But Dr. Whitman also offered two more recommendations: a chiropractor and a support group.

The chiropractor, Dr. Ed Berstein, practiced kinesiology as well and, though a relatively small man, was full of energy and exuded optimism. He had a full staff working for him and would bounce from room to room, never spending more than a few minutes with each patient.

He asked me at my first appointment to move my eyes back and forth and to stick my tongue out, but I could not accomplish either maneuver. He was obviously shocked and perplexed by my immobility, but he tried to hide it beneath an enthusiastic veneer.

"Do you really think I can get better?" I asked.

"Of course you can," he responded encouragingly.

I ended up visiting Dr. Berstein several times because I could feel the tension in my body release after each session with him. But the relief never lasted. Often the stressful forty-five minute drive back home was enough to undo his work. On top of that, we didn't see eye-to-eye on my diet or my use of prednisone and the antibiotic therapy. So I eventually stopped making appointments to see him.

My experience with a support group, meanwhile, was even less therapeutic. I had contacted the Scleroderma Foundation immediately following Dr. Whitman's initial diagnosis back in August, so I was able to refer to their literature to find a support group nearby.

Donna, not my coworker but another friend by the same name, had been calling me every day with uplifting words and hopeful wishes. She offered to drive me to the next meeting of the Mount Sinai Hospital group in New York City. I tried to refuse, telling her I didn't want to inconvenience her, but she insisted. I could go to my meeting, she said, while she ran some errands downtown.

The day of the meeting arrived, and Donna dropped me off at the hospital just as she had promised. The gathering was being held in a large conference room, where thirty or more people were seated along a pale green wall, most of them nicely dressed and – I couldn't help noticing – largely free of the deformities that had ravaged my body. I could see scleroderma in their hands and feet, but no one's illness had progressed as far as mine. I learned as we took time to introduce ourselves that most in attendance had come with a spouse or a family member. Only a small handful had come alone like me.

Several topics were covered in the meeting, including ways to cope with scleroderma, and after a guest speaker delivered a presentation on Raynaud's phenomenon, the moderator opened up the floor to those in attendance and we began sharing information and tips on medications, symptoms, and so forth.

As I sat quietly and listened, it slowly dawned on me that I had yet to hear a single sentence on the subject of healing. I had actually read about a few isolated instances of at least partial remission, but no one talked about that possibility. Instead, everyone in attendance seemed resigned to the disease and whatever course it might take, their only hope being the discovery of some miraculous cure.

Perhaps they were content to sit back and wait, I thought as I glanced around the room, but I was running out of time. Maybe someday the Scleroderma Foundation would raise enough money to fund the research to find a cure, but I would be long gone by then. I knew I was dying, but that didn't mean I had accepted it. On the contrary, I had come to the meeting looking for encouragement. Was there still hope for me? Did I still have a fighting chance?

"You shouldn't let the disease consume you," one woman in the group asserted toward the end of the meeting. "You have to go on with your life."

Her words – hopelessly Pollyannaish and nowhere grounded in what I had already experienced – finally pushed me over the edge, and I stood up to speak. "How can you say that?" I asked as I studied her perfectly normal appearance. "What are your symptoms?"

She answered that she had lost the use of a joint in the index finger on her right hand. "I have a hard time moving it," she said. On top of that, she added, she suffered Raynaud's phenomenon.

I wanted to laugh. Or cry. Instead I vented. "Hold on to that advice for people like yourself who hardly feel the effects of the disease," I seethed. "Scleroderma *has* consumed me, and I cannot just go on with my life. I can't eat. I can't sleep. I can hardly talk. My appearance has changed – and so will yours if your scleroderma progresses."

"Well," she said, trying to comfort me, "you're still the same person inside."

But I wasn't buying. "The hell I am," I objected. "I don't *feel* the same, and the world doesn't look at me the way it used to. My face and body are disfigured, and people are shocked by my appearance. I think it's very wrong for you to stand up here and just blithely tell people not to let the disease consume them." I looked around at the others. "Some of you may find you have no choice."

I sat back down, incensed by the fact that, even in a group of scleroderma victims, I was the only one who knew the sting of disfigurement – the isolation, the alienation, the emotional black hole.

I tried to shake loose my anger, but instead I found my mind drifting back to my youth in Ireland, to my bout with appendicitis while a boarding student at the Marist Convent. All by myself in the surgery ward and with no familiar faces, I had felt . . . utterly alone. Frightened to the core. I had felt the same – only more acutely – years earlier at the dispensary, where my mother had refused to chaperone me and I had been left to wait for five hours while my father ran errands in town.

And here I was again, feeling alone in a roomful of strangers, surrounded by people who didn't know me or my pain. *Same play,* I thought, *different players.*

৩৫ 13 ৩৫

Gravity, more than just a physical phenomenon, had become a powerful force in my emotional life, one that continually threatened to pull me ever lower.

After Donna picked me up at Mount Sinai Hospital and we left for home, I sat silently in the passenger's seat and pondered what I had just heard and witnessed at the support group. Somewhere between New York City and my home back in Wayne, I vowed to heal myself. I was determined to function normally again.

Moreover, as I envisioned my facial features restored – with no vestiges of disfigurement – I realized that, although it might have sounded superficial to some, my vanity would serve as my primary motivation. I would reverse the ravages of scleroderma. I would be beautiful again. Indeed, instead of gravity, I was going to answer to another of nature's forces: defiance.

If gravity was heavy, defiance was buoyant. It bubbled up from what felt like an inexhaustible wellspring of anger at my circumstances, but also from an almost surreal sense of self-confidence. I was fortunate to have Donna and Eileen and my other friends, but ultimately I realized I was alone. Nobody could go the distance with me except . . . me. I would seek help whenever and however I could, but I was ready to accept responsibility for my healing.

Of course, in the weeks and months to come, I would still encounter gravity's pull. During those low moments, I would pray for a way out of my body and my tortuous life. I had lost connection to everything I loved to do – basic and essential things like walking and talking and enjoying a good meal.

But defiance would lift me up again and again. I had discovered something within me. Like a child finding her feet beneath her for the first time, I was ready to press on, no matter how many times I fell. Part of me, in fact, was certain I would recover and that somehow, sometime I had walked this journey before, perhaps in another lifetime. I had no evidence, of course, for such a belief, just a meta-physical hunch.

At night when I slept, I dreamt I was healthy – perfectly fine – and doing all the things I'd previously taken for granted, like eating chocolate-covered macadamia nuts. In the morning, I would wake up in the same broken body, still unable to feel my numb and disfig-ured face.

But instead of being disappointed by reality, I drank from the well of defiance. I was going to beat the scleroderma. I was going to win my life back. It was only a matter of time. The dreams were an omen of good things to come.

⚭

After first being diagnosed with scleroderma, I had done some initial reading on the disease and, shocked by what I had found, had given up on knowledge in favor of denial. Some of this was healthy, I suppose. I wasn't yet ready to face my bleak prospects or imagine another, untaken road ahead.

But now, in the wake of my frustrating experiences at the sup-port group, I was ready to get my hands dirty and do some serious research. I started my quest at the Wayne Public Library, where I read every article I could find on the disease.

To my dismay, all the literature said the same thing: deformity from scleroderma was permanent. Worse still, the books and articles pointed out, remissions were rare and never permanent. Eventually, all those who fell ill with scleroderma, even those who managed to live twenty or more years after being diagnosed, eventually died from it.

Despite such bad news, I pressed on with my research, desperate to find evidence – even if it amounted to just one story – of somebody somewhere defying the odds. There had to be someone out there who had beaten the disease and reversed its deformities. As I skimmed through the books and articles, I also scanned my memories, hoping to recall a scleroderma patient I might have cared for while a nurse. Perhaps my recollections would provide some clues.

I remembered one patient, whose face looked so alien my fellow nurses and I had assumed she had endured multiple plastic surgeries. A smoker who coughed constantly, she had come to the hospital in horrible shape: poor circulation, unbearably thin. I had learned later that she did indeed have scleroderma, but my attempts to contact her family and check up on her fell short. I never found her.

The only other person who came to mind was my poor Uncle James. I vowed to beat what had consumed him.

OG

After six months on the regimen Dr. Whitman had prescribed, I was surprised to hear him declare one day in late winter that it was time to decrease my dosage of prednisone to 20mg a day. The move was a wise one, considering that the drug's potentially devastating side-effects included osteoporosis and diabetes. Long-term use was not an option.

Still, I couldn't help panicking when he announced, "I want you off the prednisone by summer."

I had grown to count on the prednisone, my lifeline to pain-free living. I couldn't imagine enduring the daily aches and pains of scleroderma without the support I knew prednisone gave to my adrenal glands. But I knew I would have to muster up the courage to try.

By the time spring arrived, I began to notice slow but perceptible changes. The color of the skin on my arms had already gone from blotchy purple to a slightly pink glow, and one day in late March after stepping out of the shower to towel off, I looked down at my ankles and noticed they, too, seemed to have taken on a more healthy pink hue. After examining them, I pinched the skin on the back of my hand and detected a hint of give.

It would be impossible to overemphasize the sheer joy I experienced upon my tiny discovery. There was hope for me.

But once again my recovery stalled. Just as it seemed my hard work might be beginning to bear fruit, I came down with what appeared to be a devastating flu. I had a sore throat, my chest was horribly congested, and I was running a high fever. Every time I coughed, I tried to expel the mucous that was multiplying in my lungs, but my hardened mouth was still so tight I couldn't open it wide enough to spit out the phlegm. I was forced to let the mucous drain slowly from the side of my mouth into a towel.

Unable to reach Dr. Whitman, who was out of town, I called Elaine Nussbaum, my macrobiotic counselor. After listening to me describe my symptoms, she suggested I might be experiencing a "healing crisis" – a condition in which the body exhibits flu-like symptoms as it expels mucous in order to cleanse itself.

After hanging up with Elaine, I called Dr. Berstein, my chiropractor, who echoed her assessment. Such a healing crisis, he said, occurred in response to various forms of healing therapies. When it occurred in response to antibiotic therapy, it was sometimes referred to as "Herxheimer Response," named after the scientist who identified the phenomenon.

While my body tried to cleanse itself, I went through an emotional exorcism as well. For three days, I was overwhelmed with grief, enduring bouts of deep, soulful crying. I could hardly move my mouth or my tongue to cry, and what came out sounded so strange and so alien to me it seemed to be coming from someone – or something – else.

I came into the kitchen one morning and, having reached rock bottom, proceeded to ignore McDuff. Normally I would have greeted him, but I was so caught up in my own misery that I didn't have the energy to bother. Suddenly I felt McDuff's tongue on the back of my leg, and I turned around and there he was, looking up at me with those big black sorrowful eyes. It was almost as if he was telling me, "It's going to be okay." It wasn't the first time – or the last – that one of our beloved dogs would contribute to my healing.

At last, when my fever broke, my mourning passed.

Bob, meanwhile, finally let me have it. He couldn't stand to see me caving in to my depression and, unable to take it any longer, informed me that he wanted out of our marriage. A terrible fight ensued, and I remember having something – I can't remember precisely what – in my right hand and wanting so badly to hit him with it but being unable even to lift my arm. He was lucky I was too weak to follow through on my impulses, because I was ready to bring the thing down on his head.

∂∂: 14 ∂∂:

Ironically, though I had been experimenting with alternative medicine for several months now, I found myself growing ever closer to my traditional caregiver, who continued to gain my trust and gratitude. Dr. Whitman had never heard of a macrobiotic diet, for instance, and often joked that he couldn't imagine life without steak and bread and all the foods I was no longer allowed to eat.

But despite his scientific background, or perhaps because of it, he was devoted not just to me and my health but also to my ideas and insights. He was open to hunches, intuition, experimentation. He didn't know much about the unconventional path I had begun to travel, but he was willing to walk it with me, to learn what he could along the way.

The relationship between doctor and patient is a complicated one, but perhaps Dr. Whitman's greatest gift was his ability to treat me like a partner, not an underling. He often wondered aloud at the wisdom of my choices, but he always respected my decisions and tried to work with me even when what I was doing worried him.

By May, I had lost nearly forty pounds, thanks to the macrobiotic diet. Dr. Whitman voiced his alarm, saying, "Your cholesterol's dropping too low on that diet. If you don't start eating differently, I'll be treating you for cancer." Cancer, he explained, had been linked to low cholesterol levels.

But I resisted his pleas. The macrobiotic diet felt right. I could sense deep down that it was helping my body heal itself.

Dr. Whitman, as usual, tried to be open to such a possibility. He had read of a report, he told me during one checkup, where Lupus-infected mice were starved and rid of their disease.

"Do you think I'm starving myself?" I asked.

"Well," he said candidly, "it *looks* like a starvation diet."

"I'm not starving," I assured him. "I can eat as much as I want."

In fact, patients taking prednisone for an extended period of time usually *gain* weight and become "pig-faced." Dr. Whitman was amazed that my weight had gone in the opposite direction.

I was certain it was the diet. I also theorized that my adrenal glands, worn out and barely functioning, were earning a much-needed rest – or were even being revitalized – thanks to the prednisone.

§

True to his word, Dr. Whitman began to wean me off the prednisone that spring. His goal was to have me completely off the steroids by summer, so the reductions came swiftly, first to 10mg a day, then to 5mg by June, then finally to zero. With each decrease, I felt a corresponding increase in discomfort, and by the time Dr. Whitman cut the dose entirely, I felt as if a host of torture-happy demons had moved into my body. The pain was crippling – and at times frightening. My sleep, restless and fitful once again, had deteriorated to nothing more than a series of twenty-minute stretches, each one punctuated by a disorienting interruption as I woke myself up with my own moaning.

Once again I felt as if I was regressing, losing whatever progress had been evident before. Walking was impossible. The pain was unbearable. And my symptoms multiplied. A calcium deposit appeared on my elbow, for which I was given a shot of antibiotics. My shoulder pain – withering enough to prevent me from raising my right arm – flared again, for which I was given a cortisone shot.

Dr. Whitman prescribed ruffin – 900mg of ibuprofen – to help alleviate the pain, but he might as well have been a medic using a small bandage to dress a gaping chest wound on the battlefield. The ruffin barely made a dent in my pain. Fortunately, I still had some prednisone stowed away, so I judiciously self-medicated when necessary. But I would need more than a small supply of quickly dwindling pills.

I found partial relief on the massage table. My first experiment with physical therapy had been cut short the previous fall after Bob had demanded I terminate the sessions with physiotherapist and family friend Diane Latteiri. But I succeeded this time around in keeping regular appointments with Nancy Waterman, a massage therapist with a home practice and someone Diane had recommended to me.

Warm and friendly, Nancy had dark hair and beautiful skin and always greeted me at her front door. Standing beside her was Sammy, her dog and a refugee from the local pound. Sammy immediately took me under his wing, often sitting outside the bedroom door and waiting while his master worked on me. For her part, Nancy, a natural nurturer, offered a soothing touch and often sent me home with a cup of warm soup, along with plenty of encouragement. I left after each session feeling uplifted, thanks not only to Nancy, who ultimately became a lifelong friend, but Sammy, whose gentle gaze always made me feel like he was hoping I'd be better the next time he saw me.

During one session with Nancy, I told her about the pain and weakness I was experiencing and shared my frustration at having regressed. She responded by suggesting I see an herbalist and gave me a recommendation for one nearby. I had never been to an herbalist before and didn't know what to expect, but I took her up on her suggestion and made an appointment.

His office, untidy and just shy of a natural disaster, looked like the sort of place where things went to get lost, and he spoke at just shy of light-speed. But I took an instant liking to the herbalist, a good-natured man who overflowed with warmth and compassion.

He introduced me to a machine with a blunt pen-sized probe, which he said was used to measure the energy flowing outward from the meridians of the body. He took my curled fingers, one by one, and showed me specific points on each one, each point corresponding to a particular internal organ. By measuring the energy at any given point, he told me, he could detect specific internal problems.

I'd never heard of such a thing during my years as a nurse, but, as had been the case before I took on a macrobiotic diet, I was open to learning something new, even if it was a little unorthodox. In fact, anything that might improve my condition seemed worth a try.

After the examination, the herbalist reported that my pituitary gland was extremely weak – at 19 instead of the normal functioning rate of 50 to 55, according to the machine he used – so he prescribed for me an herbal combination called Master Gland Formula. He also prescribed an herb called Mullin Pan Pien, which he said would help me sleep and alleviate any pain I might be having.

I was surprised to feel better after just a few days on the Master Gland Formula and the Mullin Pan Pien, which did wonders, and I couldn't help thinking back to my visit to my ailing father in Ireland in the spring of 1987. I had returned feeling worse than ever, and my instincts had pushed me to make an appointment with an endocrinologist. The capable young endocrinologist I had seen had found my thyroid functions normal after extensive testing, as had Dr. Solomon after her. But perhaps they had missed something.

Regardless, now, two years later, my hunch had been at least partially confirmed by the herbalist. The fact that I was feeling better after taking the herbal formula lent further credence to my theory. Indeed, within two weeks I was walking again – and sleeping through the night. Hoping to find refuge from my pain, I had unwittingly stumbled upon therapies for other symptoms as well.

Not long after I started feeling better, I excitedly called Elaine, my macrobiotic counselor, to tell her about the dramatic turnaround the herbs had fostered. But she responded in an uncharacteristic way.

"No, no, no, no, no herbs!" she said adamantly. "You don't combine herbs and macrobiotics. Most herbs are *very* yin, so they will disrupt the healing balance in your system."

As I listened to her speak, I told myself it would be different for me. I would do whatever I could to help ease the pain. The herbs had given me a new lease on life – new energy, new hope – not to mention at least partial freedom from the pain. As usual, I would adopt what worked. Toss what didn't. I had no interest in helping prop up whatever orthodoxy was on the line. My health was more important.

I eventually stopped seeing Elaine after she began aggressively recruiting me for her cooking classes – even though she knew I couldn't physically do the cooking and that my funds were limited.

Each health care practitioner I consulted was, not surprisingly, devoted to his or her specialty – and all the rigorously defended assumptions that went with it. Most were passionate advocates of their branch of healing; a few were charlatans.

As a patient, my job was to weed through all of the information available and find what made sense to me. My body – and its response to various treatments – provided excellent feedback, as did my intuition, my inner voice. It would take time, but I was learning to trust my instincts and to recognize my own expertise as a self-healer. I was, when it came down to it, in uncharted territory.

While I could find advice from every corner of the medical profession, mainstream or alternative, no one could offer a successful track record because no one had ever traveled beyond where I was at the moment. No patient on record, at least the record belonging to my health care providers, had fought scleroderma and lived to tell about it.

Fortunately for me, Dr. Whitman was game for the adventure. Yes, his training was in Western medicine, and his experiences traditional, but his heart and mind were open to new ideas. I felt blessed to have found a physician who understood that as a healer his job was to help me heal myself.

☿☿

As spring gave way to summer, I continued to rebound from my healing crisis and continued to make peace with life post-prednisone. I was sleeping better and managing the pain better, thanks to the herbs. My skin, too, felt softer. That landmark day back in March, when I had realized after stepping out of the shower that my body was indeed changing, had ushered in a new phase of my recovery, one that my bout with Herxheimer Response hadn't been able to stop.

But my appearance still haunted me. I had lost so much weight on the macrobiotic diet that I looked not only deformed but gaunt. Moreover, I couldn't extend my right forearm, and my hands remained curled inward. I still dreamt of one day looking healthy again, and I continued to persist with the macrobiotic diet, the herbs, and the antibiotic therapy. But I often sea-sawed between euphoria, as I noticed positive changes, and depression, as I took note of how far I had left to go. I worked things out in the quiet and solitude of our den, where I would sit and let my mind wander.

One morning while feeling rather remorseful, I followed my thoughts to an idea I had embraced several years earlier, long before I had become sick: the power of creative visualization. I don't remember precisely when the idea first took hold in my psyche, but when I was in my early twenties I watched an episode of the CBS show "60 Minutes" that supported my belief that we could actually create physical phenomenon by focusing our energy through visualization. The documentary featured several people with exceptional talents, including a Japanese boy who could project images he envisioned in his mind's eye onto film. He would close his eyes tightly as he imagined a scene, and then with a burst of energy accompanied by a sneeze or a shout, he would project the image onto the film in a Polaroid camera that sat in front of him on a table.

At one point in the documentary, a reporter asked the boy what he had visualized, and the boy answered, "Tokyo Towers," and as the television camera zoomed in on the developing Polaroid image, a faint image of the Tokyo skyline appeared.

Had it been a hoax? A staged event? As I pondered the program years later while sitting quietly in my den, I focused on a more important question: could I tap into that sort of energy and harness it for my healing? Instead of the Tokyo Towers, what if I tried visualizing myself dancing?

I did just that a few days later, setting a chair in front of me for support and closing my eyes. I imagined my feet moving . . . dancing.

My visualization sessions soon became a regular part of my morning routine. My two Westies – McDuff and Kerry – would join me in the den and take their places on the couch, where they would settle into comfortable positions and watch with their heads resting on their paws, as if to say, "Let's get going, Maureen. Entertain us!"

Little by little, after several sessions, I was able to stand without the chair. Then more progress: I was able to move my feet. *Maybe,* I ventured, *this will work*! As was the case with my morning walk, which I was still logging each day, I sometimes suffered shortness of breath and coughing and fatigue, especially when I overextended myself. But I kept at it, determined to regain my health.

Finally one morning after several months of visualizing, I found myself truly dancing.

Along with visualizing myself dancing, I created a picture in my mind's eye of my hands looking perfectly normal: slender and uncurled. I saw them folding the laundry and doing the dishes and holding onto the steering wheel. I saw them whole again.

Herbs. Massage. Visualization. I was trying anything I thought had potential – and with success – all the while diligently getting out the door each morning for my all-important walk, which was quickly becoming the foundation of my proactive recovery.

Several months went by, each one marking tiny improvements, and by November the swelling in my hands had decreased and my fingers were noticeably less curled. I was sleeping soundly now, and my joints ached less. The skin on my face was still stretched tight; thus I still looked quite disfigured, and talking still took all the energy and coordination I could muster. But I could see clear improvement. What I had envisioned was slowly coming to pass.

७ॐ 15 ७ॐ

How much of my identity had my illness claimed? Others around me no doubt had begun to associate my suffering with me, to see in my disfigured face the autoimmune disease that coursed through my blood stream. But the disease and my relationship to it ran deeper than that. It had changed more than my body. It had changed *me*. In the years to come, though I would shudder at the thought of ever reliving my encounter with scleroderma, I would come to appreciate the gift it had given me.

Yes, my body sometimes felt like my enemy, and yes, what I had thought my life should be had been stolen from me. But I could suddenly *see* things. In me. In the world around me. Because I had accepted responsibility for my own healing and because that responsibility meant leaving the well traveled path and opening myself up to new ideas previously beyond the scope of my imagination, I had changed to the core – for the better. Could I hold on to the new me?

A week before Christmas, I received news that my mother was quite ill. She had moved into a nursing home several months earlier, and I had been calling to check in on her each week. After first settling in at the nursing home, she had spent most of our early conversations complaining about the housekeepers or the food or whatnot. She had also talked a lot about all the medication she was on.

But in our last conversation, she had declared that she would not live to see Christmas. I had been annoyed at the time and had responded, "For goodness sake, don't be silly."

She had been adamant, insisting, "No, no, no. I'll be dead by Christmas." Perhaps she had known something the rest of us couldn't or wouldn't admit.

Sensing it might be my last chance to see her, I made arrangements to fly to Ireland. In fact, my gut told me something was very wrong, that this was it for my mother.

A subsequent phone conversation with my younger sister Evelyn confirmed what I had already intuited. Evelyn, who had just visited her, told me that my mother was horribly confused and that she was even talking to my father. I knew from my days as a nurse that when patients saw or spoke to the deceased, it usually meant they were about to join them.

So I got on a plane, my feet and hands still a problem but my overall health enjoying an upward arc. I dozed off not long after we cleared the runway and slept until two in the morning, when I woke up and groggily rested my face against the window. I squinted into the darkness, hoping to find the Atlantic, but could see only as far as the wispy clouds surrounding us.

Suddenly I knew my mother had died. The fact was so clear to me, and so real, that it was as if someone had just whispered into my ear the news of her death.

Evelyn was waiting for me at Dublin Airport when I arrived later that morning, and as soon as we had greeted one another she confirmed what I already knew: Mother had passed away in the middle of the night, thus fulfilling what she had predicted – that she would be dead before Christmas. I couldn't help feeling something akin to rejection. Why couldn't she have waited? The child in me felt cut short.

It had been two years since my last visit to the country of my birth, two years since I had traveled to be at my sick father's side. Now both of my parents were gone.

During my last visit, I had just begun to experience the debilitating symptoms of scleroderma. This time around, I was still wearing size eleven men's shoes, stuffed with socks to keep me warm, but I had lost so much weight I looked emaciated.

I could see the shock on Evelyn's face, but she said nothing. Nor did any of my siblings when I saw them later that day – a fact I attributed to our Irish upbringing. They all cared for me; they just didn't know how to express their concern. Moreover, I think they saw my uncle's contorted face in mine. None of them dared state the obvious, which was that they – or their children – might also be genetically primed to suffer the same fate.

We went to the hospital chapel for a burial service before the funeral, but when we arrived, the chapel was locked. We had to stand outside and wait in the bitter cold. I quickly succumbed to its chilling effects, despite the fact that I had worn three layers of socks plus woolen gloves and a hat, and I eventually grew desperate enough to duck into the emergency room to see if I could wait there until someone opened the chapel door. The young nurse on duty eyed me suspiciously, and I explained that I had just come in to get warm.

"You can't wait here," she said coldly. "This is the emergency room. You have to wait outside."

I told her I was waiting for a burial service and that I had scleroderma. "My circulation is very poor," I said. "I need to go somewhere – anywhere – out of the cold."

She remained unmoved. "You'll have to find someplace else," she said, without offering me an alternative.

I left wondering what had happened to the nursing profession. It seemed as if compassion was a skill the new generation of nurses had never learned.

Later, back at my folks' old place, I arrived with my sister and brother-in-law and was surprised to find the house much as it had been in my youth. My parents' easy chairs still sat by the fireplace, and I took a seat in my father's and reflected on my mood, which was mixed. I felt a sense of heaviness and sadness at the loss of my mother, but I also felt a sense of peace: my father and mother, married fifty years, were together again.

The rest of my siblings and cousins arrived, and we shared a meal together. To my astonishment, someone finally mentioned my condition. As my cousin Katie watched me eating only mashed potatoes – the only thing on the dinner table that I could force into my mouth – she asked, "Is that all you're eating?" She pressured me further, encouraging me to have some chicken.

Perhaps because I sensed the fear in my family, or perhaps because I simply couldn't bear to share with them what I had been through in the last two years, I didn't bother to explain my condition, responding instead, "I don't eat meat," to which Katie replied, "Oh, Jesus, Mary, and Joseph! You're goin' to shrivel up and die!"

Her words stung – because I knew I wasn't yet out of the woods and that there was a very real possibility that I might just do exactly that. Since landing in Dublin, my health had once again begun to plummet. I had been unable to continue my macrobiotic diet because I was unable to find the specials foods I needed and no one I knew owned a blender. I did the best I could, subsisting on grains and vegetables that I mashed up with a fork.

But it wasn't just my diet that was lacking. The support group I had built up around me back home was conspicuously missing. My siblings looked at me strangely, studying me with equal parts fear and curiosity. I had long since given up smoking and could no longer tolerate the smoke, but Olive, Chris – everyone smoked – and when I asked them to stop while we gathered in my parents' old kitchen, no one honored my request.

Later, while talking with Evelyn, I finally told her the name of my illness, but that was as far as it went. She didn't ask a single question about scleroderma.

At the funeral Mass, Chris sat on one side of me and Pakie Joe on the other. Numb with grief as well as the effects of scleroderma, I didn't realize that my nose was running. A girl sitting nearby handed me a tissue, and I dabbed as best I could at my tears. I couldn't feel anything, but I knew I was crying.

We went afterward into the churchyard for the burial service, and I tried to hold myself together as I greeted old friends and acquaintances. My old schoolteacher who had abused me during my childhood was there. I had sent her a letter two years earlier telling her precisely how I felt now, as an adult, about her treatment, which had haunted me all these years.

"How could you have written me a letter like that?" she demanded.

"How could I have not?" I asked.

As she walked away, I felt everything coalesce: grief for my mother, fear for my own reeling health, nostalgia for my childhood. I remembered the peace I had sensed earlier while sitting in my father's easy chair. The emotions were almost too much to bear.

As soon as the funeral was over, I knew it was time to say goodbye. I packed my things and left for Shannon Airport. It was Christmas Eve, and I was ready to go home.

❧ 14 ❧

I had been in Ireland for less than a week, but the short trip had exhausted me – emotionally and physically. I came home depleted on every level and once again fighting gravity. It was frustrating – *depressing* – to know that countless weeks of disciplined behavior and positive mental work could be undone by just a few traumatic days away from my routine.

Then one Sunday morning, less than a week after Christmas, Bob announced that he was filing for a divorce.

He was sitting at the kitchen table and reading the Sunday morning edition of The *New York Times*, his delivery as casual as it was final. "I want out of this marriage," he told me matter-of-factly. "I'm not in love with you anymore."

He went on to inform me that we didn't have what could be considered a marriage anymore and that I had changed so much that I was no longer the same person he had wed.

Then he delivered the kicker: "You don't even *look* the same."

Finally. For months I had been begging Bob to *see me* – to see my illness and how it was literally changing me, right down to my cells. And now, finally, he had grasped the truth. It was a truth I'd been living with for nearly two years, but one he couldn't face for even one more day. It was a truth I couldn't escape, but one he could cut loose while leafing through the Sunday morning paper.

I fought back tears as I tried to absorb the shock of his announcement. *How can he do this?* I thought. *How can he lose his love for me because my appearance has changed?* My mind raced as I pondered what I could have done differently. It was easy – so easy – to blame myself for the failure of our marriage. Easy, that is, until Bob inserted the last dagger.

"You know," he said caustically, "you're going to be just like your mother."

Suddenly I no longer felt like beating myself up. "No!" I protested furiously, the anger inside me building so rapidly I felt like a nuclear reactor on the verge of a cataclysmic meltdown. "I am *not* like my mother! I *married* my mother!"

Like my mother before me, I was facing a host of crippling symptoms, all of which had, until my first appointment with Dr. Whitman, been a complete mystery to me. Like her, I was fighting fear, depression, the isolation that went hand in hand with a pain no one understood. But unlike her, I had the education and the resources and the support to do something about my health. I was facing my fears, facing my illness, and I was making progress. I was doing everything I could to help heal myself.

But Bob had unwittingly stumbled upon something. Somebody in our kitchen did indeed bear an uncanny resemblance, at least on an emotional level, to my mother. Detached, unaffectionate, incapable of empathy or even sympathy – Bob shared many of my mother's shortcomings.

In that regard, he deserved my compassion, and I tried to encourage him to talk about his concerns – his fears, his pain, his insecurities – but he didn't respond. I then suggested we seek counseling to try to save our marriage, but he wanted no part of such a solution.

What he wanted, I was slowly realizing, was out of our relationship. And he wanted out fast. I suspected that financial worries were playing a part in the urgency of his desire to divorce me – he feared we would lose everything if I ended up in a nursing home – but what could I do? Though I could have never rejected my spouse over something as petty as money, I had no choice but to accept his rationale.

The next few days were spent in a daze as I wondered how I would cope with the situation. What would I say to my friends and coworkers? To my family?

I didn't have to linger long on such thoughts. Within a week I had been served with the divorce papers, which claimed I was a poor housekeeper and, because of my Catholic upbringing, a prudish and therefore incompatible lover.

I was insulted. Before my illness, I had employed a housekeeper to compensate for my busy work schedule – and the fact that I wasn't keen on housekeeping. But Bob, worried about my medical expenses and the prospect of losing our health insurance, had fired her not long after I had fallen ill. His criticism bordered on the absurd: I had been given a death sentence and was largely incapacitated by my illness, and he had fired the housekeeper – and somehow our messy house was all *my* fault (never mind his Paleolithic attitude toward housework, as if husbands were incapable of doing their fair share).

As for his claim about our sex life, that too seemed patently unfair. Certainly, as sick as I was, I was no longer interested in – or capable of – participating in an active sex life. Nor would anyone in my condition have been so inclined. Before scleroderma took over my body, I had gladly and freely entertained what I had felt was a satisfying sexual relationship. But scleroderma had stolen from me the simplest of pleasures, like eating a gourmet meal or drinking a fine wine, not to mention the ecstatic ones.

I knew Bob's grounds for divorce were hollow and superficial, that he was reneging on his vows to love me in sickness and in health. But I didn't have the energy – or the financial means – to battle him in the courtroom. I would have to let him go without a fight. Part of me wanted to find a way to do whatever I could to help salvage our marriage. Scleroderma had taught me that change, radical and pervasive, was possible. But one had to have the will to change, and I knew deep down that Bob simply wanted out of our marriage.

So I let go.

I was surprised by the freedom I felt. I didn't have much money – I was living off what I had left from my last real estate closings. But I had good credit (not to mention good credit cards), and I had faith in my ability to get by, regardless of the circumstances. I would no longer have to consult Bob about my health care or its cost, no longer have to make excuses for my macrobiotic diet or apologize for the unpleasant aroma. Bob didn't like the smell of seaweed boiling on the stove. But I no longer minded it. And I was the only person I had to please now.

❦ 17 ❦

Nineteen-ninety began an awful lot like the year before it. I told Dr. Whitman at an appointment in January that once again I was struggling. Tight, hard skin. Swollen feet and hands. Sore joints. All of my recent progress seemed in jeopardy now, thanks in no small part to the one-two-punch that came in the form of my mother's death and the death of my marriage. The emotional weight of those back-to-back blows felt like more than I could bear. My physical state, already precarious, reeled from the dual impact. I was ready for more help.

While it's true I didn't begin to heal until I took full responsibility for my health, it's also true that, as much as I had to go it alone, I would need – and had already graciously accepted whenever it had arrived – help along the way. Consider it one of the many paradoxes of my recovery: I was alone, yet sometimes it felt as if people like Dr. Whitman and Nancy Waterman had been sent to me, as if someone or something in the universe was looking out for me.

And then there was Anthony Folari. If Dr. Whitman and the others had been delivered to me, Anthony was nothing short of an angel. I had never seen anyone so radiant – almost *transparent* – as Anthony, an Italian-American who, with his dark hair, brown eyes, and beautiful, easy smile, exuded honesty and integrity. His face shone, as if expressing an inner light.

I met him while standing in an aisle at my health food store on a cold January afternoon. (I would later meet his wife, who was also extraordinary; together they made a beautiful young couple.) Gentle and polite, almost serene in his mannerisms, Anthony struck me as especially trustworthy, and I immediately found myself deep in a conversation with him about my ongoing battle with scleroderma.

When I told him I had been experimenting with nontraditional medicine and that I was open to new ideas, he suggested I look into iridology. He wasn't a doctor or for that matter an expert on the subject, he told me, but he had studied iridology with Dr. Bernard Jenson, a well-known chiropractor and nutritionist.

I had never heard of iridology, and I listened with a keen interest as Anthony described the process of taking photographs of a patient's eyes to diagnose physical problems throughout his or her body. I was intrigued and asked Anthony if he would take photographs of my eyes and review the results with me.

"I don't think so," he said bashfully. "I'm not a doctor or even a nutritionist."

Undeterred, I pressed him on the matter until he agreed, although he insisted on providing the service for free.

We met a few days later at his apartment for what would turn out to be the two most enlightening hours of my life. I learned the fundamental tenet of iridology – that each part of the iris can indicate the condition of a corresponding internal organ – and recognized it mirrored the same principle elucidated by my herbalist, which was that my fingertips could provide clues about the health of my internal organs.

After taking several photographs of my irises and analyzing them, Anthony met me for a follow-up meeting to discuss the results. I was tired and cold and felt awfully weak when I arrived at his apartment, and Anthony responded by tenderly preparing me a cup of tea – in the microwave, which I found quite amusing. We then sat down to study the photographs in what turned out to be a lengthy session.

Anthony identified significant problems with my lungs, colon, liver, and skin and suggested I do a seven-day colon cleanse. He referred me to a handful of books on healing by Dr. Jenson, but after starting one of the doctor's books, I immediately put it down. The information presented – particularly the content of the images – was sobering in its graphic detail. I told myself I would come back to the subject when I felt stronger.

ॐ

In fact, although my body was one of my chief concerns at the time, I was more concerned about my mind. I was still grieving my mother's death as well as my divorce, and I knew I should be seeking counseling to help me sort through the many issues I was facing.

My divorce from Bob wasn't legal yet (it would take months for the paperwork to go through), and he and I had decided to continue sharing the house for the foreseeable future. (I would buy him out years later.) Our divorce had taken some of the pressure off our relationship in some ways, but the specter of our failed marriage still hung over us, and cohabitating with him made moving on emotionally a bigger challenge than it already was.

On top of all that, money remained an issue. My illness had left me in a Catch 22: I had to rest to recover, but I had to work to pay for my recovery and all of the expensive remedies in my regimen.

Fortunately for me, I found a good listener in my priest, who agreed to supplement my paid counseling sessions with sessions of our own.

Father John Connell, ever patient and not without a sense of humor, might have reconsidered had he been able to divine our first session, during which I ranted on about how much I disliked the Catholic Church and the clergy. Afterward he told me I would have made a good Hindu. But he stuck with me, and in the weeks to come he let me vent about my marriage and my situation at home and all the anger I was experiencing.

Somewhere along the line, I began to talk about saving my marriage. I wanted Bob to get counseling, and I wanted to do whatever I could to right the sinking ship that was our relationship. But it was a fleeting hope. Bob wanted out. He had told me as much that Sunday after Christmas, and nothing had changed.

Father Connell, smart enough to know a lost cause when he saw one, advised me to let my marriage go. "Imagine yourself holding two pink balloons," he suggested one day. "Pink is the color of peace. Imagine Bob inside one balloon and yourself inside the other. Then, take a pair of scissors and cut the string attached to the balloon that holds Bob and let it fly off into the sky. Watch it peacefully drift out of sight."

It was a handy visualization technique. But it didn't work for me at first. Instead, I repeatedly resisted the image of letting go of Bob's balloon. I couldn't face the bleak finality of saying good-bye to my marriage.

When I wasn't feeling resistant, I was feeling spiteful. Instead of imagining what Father Connell had suggested, I imagined stabbing Bob's balloon with the scissors and watching him crash to the earth.

Eventually, though, after imagining countless variations on the theme, I cut Bob loose.

捠

With that piece of work done, it was time to revisit another demon – a drastic, disgusting demon. It was time to follow through on Anthony's recommendation of an internal cleansing. My first foray into the topic had been a brief and unsettling one, but I had since drummed up enough courage to finish Dr. Jenson's book and had found his theories credible. Indeed, it made sense that a lifetime of poor eating habits and troubled digestion could all too easily lead to an inhospitable environment in the colon and that a thorough cleansing could improve the digestive processes.

By now I was seeing Dr. Whitman only once a month, and I had weaned myself from most of my medications. My condition had improved, but the disease hadn't gone into remission. I still looked deformed, still experienced continual fatigue – thus I was still ready to try almost anything to beat the scleroderma. I knew enough of what was to come, though, to be frightened. I had seen the photos in Dr. Jenson's book. I had read the accounts. I would be pumping several gallons of water through my intestines – and dealing with the filthy fallout of such a radical procedure.

With the help of an appendix in Dr. Jenson's book, I found the number of a company that sold a colema set and ordered one, which arrived with a five-gallon enema apparatus, cleansing agents like bentonite clay and psyllium, and supplements like potassium, niacin, calcium, chlorella, and wheat grass powders. The colon cleansing protocol was intimidating, not to mention time-consuming: I was to eat no solid food for six days, during which I was to perform various tasks in conjunction with the cleansing every one to two hours.

Bob thought I was nuts – and told me so in no uncertain terms, informing me that what I was doing was the most abnormal thing he'd ever witnessed. But he built a bench for me to sit on in the bathroom and helped me fill the bags with water.

"I think you're losing it," he would say as he huffed upstairs with another five-gallon bag of water.

"No," I quipped, "I'm losing something, but not my head."

"Did you talk with your doctor about this?" he asked, dumbfounded.

"Yes," I lied.

I stuck with the protocol, and after six days of fasting and cleansing, I felt utterly, thoroughly exhausted. I was so weak I could hardly talk. But within just a few days of finishing the cleanse I noticed a radical shift in my energy: it soared.

I wanted to rush into Dr. Whitman's office with the results of my latest outlandish experiment, but I hesitated. Dr. Whitman would often begin our appointments by saying, "So, Maureen, what crazy stuff are you trying now?" I was certain when he heard about the colon cleanse he would think I had finally gone over the edge.

But he surprised me once again. He listened attentively and took careful notes, afterward stuffing them into my file, which by now took up two folders.

∽∾

Funny thing about energy: the more you have, the more you want. Since those first groggy mornings years earlier when I had forced myself out of bed and into the real estate office, I had been watching my vigor steadily disappear. It had begun to feel like what little energy I had left could travel only one way: out. But the colon cleanse had given me a taste of what it was like to truly feel alive. I felt invigorated and I was eager for more.

I asked Anthony in our next meeting about other methods that might increase my energy and continue to feed my euphoria, and he suggested wheatgrass juicing. Once again refusing any compensation, he educated me on the benefits of the technique which, like my macrobiotic diet, promised to deliver wholesome, nutrient-packed fuel at less cost than processed food. Advocates of wheatgrass juicing claimed it could counteract toxins and carcinogens in the body, improve digestion, reduce high blood pressure, prevent tooth decay – even aid in the prevention and cure of cancer.

If it had a downside it was purportedly the taste, which not surprisingly resembled . . . grass. But countless longtime fans and recent converts had learned to like it – or mask it by blending it with juice – in order to reap the benefits of consuming several amino acids, plus vitamins A, B, C, and E care of one small straight shot of the stuff. The final product, homegrown and served fresh, was seventy percent chlorophyll, the nutrient behind photosynthesis.

After investing in several startup supplies – including an expensive wheatgrass juicer – I diligently planted the wheatgrass seeds into shallow trays of soil and placed the trays near my kitchen windows, where they made an instant indoor garden. As soon as the seeds had grown into vibrant green grass, I began harvesting the wheatgrass for my juicing therapy.

My first shot of the stuff was fairly uneventful, mainly because by now my taste buds were hardly functioning. What I could taste wasn't particularly appealing, but it went down pretty easy for two reasons. To begin with, drinking wheatgrass juice took me back to my childhood, when we used to pluck what we called "long grass" from the fields and chew on the ends of it. Secondly, part of my healing I owed to a newfound sense of courage: I would swallow a frog, I told myself, if it helped me beat scleroderma. I was willing to do whatever it took to speed my recovery, including toughening up what was left of my taste buds.

Along with wheatgrass, I also sprouted sunflower seeds, clover, and alfalfa. I had never tended a garden before, and growing my own gave me a remarkable sense of power. Moreover, I discovered a connection between the tiny seeds germinating in my kitchen garden and my own healing. Suddenly, I had become aware – acutely aware – of the healing that was going on around me every second of every day. I had become an active and creative agent in the revitalization of my body.

By the end of spring, I noticed what I had been told was impossible: my hands had begun to uncurl. I visited Dr. Whitman in June and showed him the undeniable evidence.

"See!" I said excitedly. "My hands are straightening out!" I then asked what was foremost on my mind. "Do you think my face will ever return to normal?"

"Well," he said solemnly, "that would be a miracle."

I looked at him defiantly. "Well, I believe in miracles."

I truly did. But like anyone clinging to a faith in the unseen, I still had misgivings. I would have never guessed that a voice on a cassette tape could erase those lingering doubts.

֍

You're not in the world. The world is in you.

I wish I could claim such a grand idea as my own, but the insight belongs to the popular author and spiritual guru Dr. Depak Chopra. I came across it while listening to a tape of one of his best-selling books, *Unconditional Life*.

Chopra's words – calming and reassuring – solidified my belief that I could completely heal, and his ideas prompted me to see the universe in a fundamentally different way. As I listened to his encouraging voice, I felt so connected to his revelations that I felt as if he had made the tape especially for me. In fact, I made myself *believe* he had made the tape for me because the image helped me experiment with the vast energetic connections his work suggested we could harness through our imaginations.

My relationship to Chopra and his wisdom was anything but passive. I practiced his ideas, putting them to work for me, and I followed one of his suggestions while meditating by letting my thoughts flow without conscious direction from my intellect.

For the next several months, I carried the tape with me as if it were a life-saving antidote to a deadly poison. I listened to it as I greeted the morning, listened to it in my car as I ran errands during the day, listened to it at night before drifting off to sleep. Each session fed my creative powers and strengthened my resolve. I had found someone whose belief in infinite possibilities mirrored my faith in miracles. Why couldn't I heal fully? What could possibly stop me if I threw everything I had into my recovery?

"Listen to the one who is listening," Chopra intoned. His words formed a potent refrain that countered the noise daily swirling in my head: the negative feedback, the crippling doubts, the creeping cynicism that wanted nothing more than to swallow me whole.

I had been trying for months to meditate, but *I* had been the one asking all the questions, *I* had been the one guiding every reflection. The constant chatter – I still struggle to shut it down to this day. But until then, I had never realized how much it ran me or how badly my mind craved quiet.

Who was listening?

I hadn't paid much attention. Until now.

ஐ 18 ஐ

Who *was* listening? Before playing the tape of *Unconditional Life*, I had never bothered to ask such a question. But there was someone – something – out there. *In here*. Listening. Call it what you will – Allah, Jesus Christ, Karl Jung's "collective unconscious," the inner wisdom that is beyond yet within all of us – I didn't care to name it. I had stumbled upon enough truth for me: there was power in healing – untapped and limitless. And that power belonged to everybody, including me.

I had adopted one of Chopra's mantras: pure being, saying to itself, "Become the water," becomes the water. I would repeat the saying over and over in my mind as I drifted off to sleep each night, all the while knowing I had the power to change my whole world.

I had escaped Dr. Whitman's dire prognosis. But I wanted to do more than survive. If I had been granted more time on this earth, I was going to make the most of it.

I continued meditating, continued reshaping how I viewed the universe and my place in it, and by the following summer, the summer of 1991, I realized my worst days were behind me. Scleroderma had given me its best shot, and I was still standing. In fact, I was walking a mile each day and enjoying every step, every breath, both of which were coming easier now. I was still on antibiotics and still taking the Armour thyroid, but otherwise was living drug-free. My energy and outlook showed vast improvement.

But my contorted face, specifically my mouth, still hindered day-to-day living. Chewing was still a laborious ordeal, complete with drooling, whether I was choking down another liquid meal or trying my luck at solid food.

Just as troubling, my range of motion was severely limited. Though I was walking every day, I was about as limber as a pretzel – and about as coordinated as a punch-drunk prizefighter. The only way I could have made it across a balance beam would have been on my stomach.

After listening to me describe my problems with balance and coordination, Anthony Folari asked me if I had tried yoga. The exercises, he told me, helped people with subtle muscle control, something I didn't possess.

I didn't have much money to spend on a yoga course, so I decided to sit in on the weekly class offered at the local high school. But my first foray into yoga was discouraging: I couldn't move as easily as the other students, and I had difficulty doing even the most basic movements, like lying on my back and bringing my knees up to my chest. The mobility in my right arm and shoulder was still restricted, and my bones still felt sore. I couldn't keep up with the class and felt embarrassed that I couldn't execute the instructor's simplest of commands. I quit the class – without regret or shame. I knew I would find my way.

In fact, I found Michelle Kouri, a private yoga instructor in nearby Demarest. Tall and thin, with deep-set hazel eyes and a head-hugging crew cut, Michelle boasted a hearty laugh and a serene yet fun-loving demeanor. I liked her immediately.

She listened attentively as I explained my first encounter with yoga and detailed my health and flexibility problems, and then we went to work. But to my surprise, we didn't start with movements, postures, or stretches but with breathing. It seemed an odd thing to practice, considering I'd been breathing all my life without ever thinking about it. But when Michelle explained that the first priority of yoga was breath control and started demonstrating the technique, I realized that I had never known how to breathe properly. I wasn't alone, Michelle assured me. Most people didn't know how to do so.

Most people, though, had at least some semblance of flexibility. As soon as we started in with the actual movements, my deficiencies took center stage. I couldn't kneel because of the stiffness in my knees, and I couldn't sit back on my heels because of the tightness in my thigh muscles.

Michelle gently assisted each movement, manipulating my arms and legs into the proper positions while I focused on breathing. Call it *assisted yoga*. With Michelle at my side, I managed to work my way into each posture, slowly, gently, gingerly, and it dawned on me that gravity wasn't the only force I had been contending with these last few years; atrophy, too, had taken a toll on my health. Yoga promised to awaken my long-dormant muscles.

My first session with Michelle was so positive and nurturing that I decided to make it a weekly affair. I looked forward to each visit, which soon grew into something more than mere exercise. While she taught me the movements, she also elicited my feedback. How was I feeling physically and emotionally? How was my ongoing recovery progressing? I felt instantly calm in her presence. Sometimes just hearing her laugh – her deep, hearty laugh – would uplift my spirits for the entire day.

Michelle had been teaching yoga for years, but despite her experience, I think she found in me an unprecedented challenge. Every time I would attempt to breathe from my abdomen, my face would tighten. And every time I tried to engage my muscles, I would panic. But Michelle quickly developed ways to help me overcome my fears. Over time it seemed as if she not only saw me but could *sense* me. On more than one occasion she had her back to me but still managed to catch me tensing up.

"Relax your face," she would say soothingly. "You've tightened it again."

Along with encouraging me to envision a disease-free future, Michelle helped me live in the present. When I confessed that the yoga exercises sometimes felt painful, she told me to be in the pain.

"Be in the moment and accept where you are right now," she encouraged me.

Opening up physically after having closed down for so many years overwhelmed and frightened me. It seemed as if I clung to the tightness – to the scleroderma – because in some ways it had protected me. Like a knight who had worn protective clothing for a battle that was now over, I had to learn that it was safe to shed my armor.

Michelle eventually helped me develop a daily yoga routine, which began every morning as soon as I woke up. I would sit on the edge of my bed and breathe deeply, using my abdomen and diaphragm. Michelle had taught me to pull in my abdomen muscles while pressing my chest forward, which helped keep my chest expanded. Each time I did this exercise, I hooked my thumbs under my arms like the old suspenders-wearing farmers on the 70s-era television show "Hee Haw." Then I would rise out of my sitting position on the edge of the bed to do a series of beautiful yoga stretches in a standing position, bowing to honor the sun. My sun salutation was far from perfect – my poses barely resembled the textbook examples – but I felt calm and centered when I performed the exercises.

I practiced yoga every morning, after which I would leave for my morning walk. When I came back inside, I would finish with some more yoga stretches, lying on the floor and stretching my arms out to open the areas of my chest where my muscles were their tightest.

As the weeks went by and I continued with my exercises, I began to develop a new awareness of my body. I noticed when I was tensing up or breathing shallowly or letting my daily routine lose its natural balance. Like my meditation practice and the insights I had gleaned from my Depak Chopra tape, yoga helped me connect my body to my emotions and to my spirituality. I began to realize that the constricted skin and the atrophied muscles in my body reflected my resistance to life, my fear of letting go, my need to control things beyond my control. I had closed myself off, but yoga, thanks to Michelle's mentorship, could help me learn to open up again.

Scleroderma didn't have to be a death sentence. It could be a powerful catalyst for change.

೦೦

The more open I became to transformative experiences, the more easily they came to me. The more I stretched myself, the less confined I felt in my own skin. Scleroderma had chipped away at my life, carving away every comfort, everything known, while leaving me an alien in my own body. Like an ever-tightening circle, it had slowly but steadily consumed everything that made me who I was. Had it continued unchecked, it would have been all that remained in the end. But I had found a way out.

Freedom, I was learning, meant following the adventure of my recovery wherever it went. One day in December I stopped in at a health food store in Ridgewood, not my normal haunt, and overheard Ed, the store's owner, talking with a customer about magnetic therapy. A tall, thin man in his mid sixties, Ed was recovering from prostate cancer. He had traveled overseas to a clinic in Germany to receive the experimental treatment.

I had heard about magnetic therapy but had never investigated it, so it seemed as good a time as any to find out more. I asked Ed for a quick tutorial on the subject, and he told me magnets had two poles – one positive and the other negative – and that some doctors prescribed the use of negative magnetic polarity to help people heal. He then referred me to a book on the subject written by Dr. William H. Philpot, a retired physician who had used magnetic therapy in his medical practice for more than forty years.

I bought Dr. Philpot's book, read it cover to cover, and then called him at his office in Oklahoma. He quizzed me about my health, running down a specific set of questions as he did, and I answered each one as thoroughly as I could. When I told him that I was extremely sensitive to computers and televisions, he explained that I was probably magnetically deficient. Many people suffered from sensitivities like mine, he said, because the magnetism of the earth had been compromised by the electromagnetic fields associated with modern technology. He suggested I try sleeping on specially designed magnets that he sold to his patients.

Not surprisingly, the magnets were expensive, so I bought only as many as I could afford: ten of them, each measuring three inches wide by six inches long by one-half inch thick. Following Dr. Philpot's instructions, I placed each magnet between a piece of egg-crate foam and my mattress, with the negative pole facing upward and the positive side facing the floor.

My first night of sleeping on them was pure bliss: I slept through the night and awoke feeling energized. I felt so convinced they had made a significant difference that I used a credit card to purchase the full set of twenty-four magnets to cover the entire surface of my bed. I didn't regret the decision.

Within a few months of sleeping on the magnets, my shoulders had un-hunched, and I felt positively youthful. I even bought a set for McDuff, who was twelve now and lame. His amazing recovery – in four weeks, x-rays by our veterinarian showed McDuff's arthritis had actually reversed – made it into Dr. Philpot's lectures.

Meanwhile, I couldn't wait to share the results at my next appointment with Dr. Whitman.

"So, Maureen," he said as he took a seat across from me in the examination room, "what crazy stuff are you doing now?"

"Well," I said coyly, "I'm sleeping on a bed of magnets."

Dr. Whitman doubled over in his chair in a fit of gut-busting laughter. I'd never seen him laugh so hard. "So you're sleeping on magnets now!" he mused and shook his head in disbelief.

He straightened up as soon as I told him how convinced I was that the magnets were healing my joints and expediting my recovery. Whether or not he believed such an idea, he dutifully jotted down my explanation, adding another page to the reams of notes that comprised my file while treating my report with an open yet critical inquisitiveness.

I wasn't the only one with news to share. Dr. Whitman informed me after my latest round of blood work came in that my antinuclear antibody had come down significantly – from a dilution of 1/5,500 to 1/320. But I hadn't reached my goal of a normal count (between zero and fifty). As for my sedimentation rate, it was still fluctuating between thirty and thirty-five, still above the normal range of zero to twenty, but not off the charts.

Overall, Dr. Whitman was quite pleased – not to mention surprised – by my progress. But my latest results showed an increase in a particular type of enzyme that usually indicated the potential for liver damage, thanks in this case to my long-term use of antibiotics. After three years on doxicycline, it was time to call it quits. As had been the case when Dr. Whitman told me he would be weaning me off prednisone, I wondered how I would get by without antibiotics.

But, unlike my painful farewell to prednisone, this one was uneventful. I was ready for the change.

ꙮ 19 ꙮ

Despite – or perhaps because of – my traditional Catholic upbringing, I no longer considered myself a religious person. Spiritual, yes. But religious, no. Though I was still devoted to certain elements of the Catholic faith and still attended Mass on occasion, I was happy to cede the dogmatic underside of my childhood creed – eternal damnation and such – to the Church. I was finding my own path, one that viewed this life in mystical terms: the body was a shell and only a small part of who we were. Like a computer screen, it reflected a bigger reality that was going on inside: energy.

Ever since Dr. Whitman had first diagnosed my illness, I had been finishing each day the same way: as I closed my eyes to fall asleep, I prayed that when I woke up in the morning I would look in the mirror and find my face fully restored. Night after night, I prayed for the same miracle. And morning after morning, I awoke to the same disappointment. I was still sick. Still disfigured.

By the spring of 1992, a slow accumulation of small changes had amounted to huge gains. But my healing was still incomplete. I still had the face of a woman scarred by scleroderma. It was time to try another alternative healing therapy.

I had read a few articles over the years on an unconventional healing technique called "rebirthing," which sought to liberate a person from their painful past in order to hasten a full recovery from whatever it was that ailed them. The net effect was akin to a second birth, albeit a spiritual or emotional one. Could it work for me?

There was only one way to find out.

After noticing an ad for rebirthing in a health magazine, I called the number, and a man named John answered. I told him my story, and John, a rebirthing practitioner who lived in New York City, explained the rebirthing process more fully.

I made an appointment for June 12, the day before my fiftieth birthday. I kept my appointment a secret, despite my fears of visiting a complete stranger in his apartment in the city. What I was about to undertake would likely raise a few eyebrows, and I didn't need any negative feedback – I was getting enough internally. A voice inside me warned, "You must be crazy to do this without telling anyone where you're going." But I ignored it.

I felt my heart in my throat when John, a burly man with a kind face, opened the door to his dimly lit upstairs apartment and invited me inside. His greeting was warm, but his apartment was a bit dark. As he closed the door behind me, I spotted a huge black cat watching me with vibrant green eyes.

"How do you feel about being here?" John asked.

"Well," I said cautiously, "I have to tell you I'm a little bit nervous."

"I thought you would be," he said and then explained what we were about to do. By lying down comfortably on the floor and using a series of connected breaths, he told me, I could reach an altered state of consciousness that would allow me to bring up old memories and release myself from them. Without further explanation, he suggested we begin.

He led me to a small futon, which rested on the floor, and instructed me to lie down on my back with my hands at my side. He then sat down on a cushion beside me to coach me through a series of breaths.

"Breathe in from your abdomen," he said calmly, "and bring it all the way up to the clavicle, and then, with one circular expression, connect it to your exhalation, bringing it back down through your torso."

I did as he instructed, breathing through my mouth as I did, and within a short time I felt as if my body had turned to stone. I had lost feeling in my face, my hands, my feet. I felt a shiver run through me – I was as cold as ice – and I panicked.

He could sense my fear and told me to keep breathing, to breathe through the fear, but I barely heard him. *This is it*, I thought. *I'm going to die. I'm finished.* I was a frozen statue: rooted to the futon and shackled by my own fear.

John's voice barely broke through the fog. "Keep breathing," he urged me. "Keep breathing."

I did as he said, but suddenly I was afraid to open my eyes, as if I might not be there when I opened them, as if I had already died.

Keep breathing.

I no longer heard John's voice; I *felt* it inside my head. Slowly, imperceptibly at first, my terror disintegrated, until all that was left was a growing sense of peace, a rose blooming in the desert.

At the center of that peace, for a fleeting instant, as if frozen on a movie frame, the face of an infant appeared before me. I gazed at the baby girl and instantly recognized myself in her face. *How could I have forgotten how beautiful she was?* I asked myself. *How could I have forgotten her sense of joy, her sense of wonder?* I was sobbing now, over-whelmed by the memory. *I was beautiful when I entered this world. I was perfect.*

The image disappeared, and I found myself back at John's dark apartment, with him coaching me back to consciousness, to normal breathing. After about ten minutes, I sat up slowly and found myself filled with joy. I had connected with a long-lost part of myself – a radiance I'd buried in my subconscious – and I knew already that I had unlocked doors that would speed my healing. The tightness, the numbness, the self-critical expression on my face – all could be traced to the fears I was afraid to let go. Just as scleroderma had restricted my physical movement, my self image had held me in spiritual bond-age. I had buried the real me – my authentic self – by suppressing my emotions and their rightful expression. I had been wearing a mask, but rebirthing had torn it free, giving me a brief glimpse of my true, perfect self. I had found the courage to love myself unconditionally.

☙☙

I made an appointment to return the following week, but found my second session relatively uneventful. Still encouraged, I made a third appointment so I could explore the process further.

The terrible fear returned at the third session, but now I trusted it: I knew it served a purpose. I allowed myself to breathe into and through it, and as the session proceeded I felt myself drift in and out of little pockets of fear. I kept at the breathing technique, continuing to connect my inhalation to my exhalation in a circular breathing pattern, and I sensed my past merging with the present. By the end of the session I felt relaxed – so relaxed I nearly fell asleep – and in the space between waking and sleeping another extraordinary thing happened: someone spoke to me as if in a dream, saying, "Go with the universe, not against it."

After eight more sessions John invited me to an underwater rebirthing ceremony at a private home on the Jersey shore. I had never been much of a swimmer and I felt leery about getting into the pool, but after some coaching from John I donned nose plugs, earplugs, and a snorkel and submerged myself.

I was surprised to experience an even more profound letting go underwater than I had achieved at John's apartment. The sense of peace was exhilarating, not to mention addictive, and I didn't want to leave the pool once we were through.

Happily, I was elated to find that, even after getting out of the water and dressing to go home, the peaceful feeling remained. I felt it in my face and in my skin, which suddenly felt soft and relaxed. When I shared my gratitude with John, he suggested I bring the nose plugs, earplugs, and snorkel with me into the bathtub at home some-time and try to emulate the process alone. I did – often – and found it quite soothing.

It wasn't long before I discontinued my appointments with John. I had learned what rebirthing could teach me: to take responsibility for releasing myself from the inner prison I had created by living in fear. Just as important, I realized now that there was a place to go in my meditations, a place to go to heal the essence of me. I would seek out the little girl inside me and give her whatever she needed to grow in health and wisdom.

ΘΘ

The little girl – she was like a ghost. Ephemeral, elusive, she came and went as she pleased. After finishing my rebirthing sessions, I began the work of visualizing the little girl, trying to bring her back while meditating.

My daily routine now included up to twenty circular rebirthing breaths, which helped me focus on my heart instead of my head. I envisioned the child and searched for ways to communicate with her, but I found it difficult to see her face as clearly as I'd seen it during my first rebirthing session. When I did see her face, I couldn't hold onto the image. Sometimes she appeared spontaneously without beckoning, while at other times no amount of effort on my part could elicit an appearance. Days and sometimes weeks went by without her, no matter how hard I tried to conjure up a visit – she had been locked away for so long. But I persisted in trying to make contact with her. I knew that eventually my patience would pay off. One day she would feel safe enough to speak to me.

Sometimes while meditating I would invite the little girl to voice her feelings. As I did, a judgmental voice inside would say in an accusing tone, "What? Are you crazy or something? Hearing voices?" But I pressed on. Yes, what I was doing was unconventional, enough so that it made me feel self-conscious. But my intellect would have to idle its engines for a while. It was time to follow my heart.

At other times, when I did see the child, she was crying quietly with her head hanging down and her shoulders hunched over. I knew I had to get her to trust me, and during each meditation I would silently ask her to tell me what she needed, but she never responded.

Finally one morning I tried a different approach. I began by admiring her looks and praising her. As I did, I began to feel the numbness in my face recede and the energy in my body change, relax.

"You're beautiful," I told her. "You can trust me."

Some people pay psychotherapists to facilitate this kind of dialogue, but I no longer had enough money to pay an expert. Nor did I have health insurance that would cover sessions with a therapist. In fact, I had no health insurance at all by the time I began meditating on my child-self. I was in scary territory – walking a low-budget tightrope without a safety net – but I felt strangely confident. I was rebuilding myself from the inside out. Money and security – i.e., returning full-time to work – could wait.

I took at least twenty minutes every morning after breakfast and my walk to sit in meditation, invoking the child's voice, coaxing her to speak to me. I knew that when she finally spoke, it would symbolize the recovery of a part of me I had lost so long ago. The other voice – the judgmental, doubting one – insistently countered my desire to sit in meditation.

"Don't you have work to do?" it would say in a condescending tone. "Why are you sitting around doing nothing?"

It took courage to sit in silence, but listening had become my mission. I was determined to make contact with the part of me that had shut down. What had been self defense during my childhood was impeding my growth as an adult.

Many of the books I read at the time suggested meditating for twenty minutes in the morning and then for the same amount of time again in the evening, but my meditations were frequent – and often long.

As with so many of the other therapies I tried, I altered the textbook advice to suit my needs. I usually began my meditations by instructing my face to relax. Then I consciously moved the relaxation down my body. By the time my focus reached my abdomen, my face had usually tightened again, so I would start over. I never thought of giving up. Instead, every time I noticed even a trace of relief from the constant tightness in my face, I closed my eyes and visualized the child.

Slowly I realized I had to put on that little girl's face and relive her childhood. I had to give her all that she had been denied – unconditional love, admiration, protection. I meditated for months, but she never spoke to me. Yet I sensed she was beginning to trust me because in my meditations I occasionally saw her smile. As I envisioned her, memories from my childhood poured forth. One in particular came vividly to mind.

I was back in grade school, sitting in the Spartan schoolroom where the heat from the fire went straight up the chimney, and my abusive teacher was once again ridiculing me. I was sobbing, overwhelmed by a terrible sense of shame.

As I continued to meditate, I gave myself what I had needed that day. I put my arms around my child self and comforted her. I gave her a tissue for her tears, smoothed her hair, and held her close. I asked her what she wanted to say about the teacher who had been so cruel to her, and she confessed she almost wanted to kill her.

I told her it was all right to feel that way and then closed the meditation while holding her close to me.

Love would conquer fear.

❧ 20 ❧

I t was back. The recurring dream that had haunted me before my
illness had resurfaced during my recovery, evolving along with my
health. Once again, the waves chased me as I slept. Years earlier, I had
dreamt more than once that I had succumbed to the waves, each time
waking with a start just before drowning.

Now I played with the dreams while meditating. I let the water
wash over me, bathing me rather than drowning me. Instead of
destructive force, I gave the ocean healing power. Instead of surren-
dering, I created something new.

Meditation, I was slowly realizing, had unleashed in me a powerful creative energy. As I exercised that energy, I often felt frightened
and guilty. The God defined by the Catholic Church of my youth
was a jealous one, a wrathful one – and certainly not one to welcome
me as a co-creator. Learning to meditate meant learning to outgrow
such a tiny deity. But such a feat was possible outside the narrow
confines of my upbringing. Other people had learned to tap into
their own power, their own sacred connection to the universe. Why
couldn't I?

A public television program entitled *Healing and the Mind,* hosted
by journalist Bill Moyers, prompted me to investigate the practice
of T'ai Chi, which Moyers profiled in depth while documenting

the relationship between the mind and body in healing. T'ai Chi, an ancient Chinese art that combines meditation with movement, immediately appealed to my thirst for new knowledge of myself and my healing.

I began my exploration of T'ai Chi by attending a class at a nearby martial arts academy, where about forty people were gathering. While the students enthusiastically found their places and readied themselves for what appeared to be a well-practiced routine, I looked around the packed room and wondered if I was out of my league. My fears multiplied when the class started and the instructor began leading a series of exercises I couldn't follow.

I listened intently, but, as had been the case during my first experiment with yoga, I couldn't do even the simplest moves correctly. When the instructor relayed a basic command such as, "Raise your right arm," I found myself raising my left. It was as if a short circuit existed somewhere between my brain and the rest of my body. I felt stymied by my lack of coordination and balance. *If this is T'ai Chi,* I thought, *forget it! I'm never going to make it through.*

I never went back to the academy, and I temporarily abandoned the idea of learning T'ai Chi. But the motivation to learn returned to me the following spring, in 1993, when I saw an ad in the paper for a course in a gentler form of T'ai Chi called T'ai Chi Chih. Chilton Memorial Hospital in Pompton Plains, a town bordering Wayne, had run the ad, and I called the hospital to sign up for the class, which wasn't scheduled to begin until October.

I enrolled anyway and eagerly arrived at the hospital that fall for my first shot at learning T'ai Chi Chih. I stepped inside the chapel, where the class was held, and was chagrined to find not one person in attendance under the age of seventy, save for our instructor, a nun wearing her habit. *Boy, am I in the wrong place!* I thought. But I joined the circle they made toward the front of the chapel and listened as Sister Antonia introduced herself.

A little plump but possessing great charm, Sister Antonia had a youthful face, snow-white hair, and beautiful blue eyes. As she spoke, she exuded serenity and a joyful temperament, and I suddenly felt at utter ease in her presence.

How strange, I mused, that a Catholic nun was about to lead an exercise in an ancient Chinese art. The nuns of my youth would have never dreamt of exploring, much less sharing, an Eastern tradition.

As soon as she finished with her opening remarks, Sister Antonia went around the circle and asked each student why he or she had come to the class. When my turn came, I told Sister Antonia and the class about my struggle with scleroderma and about the different healing methods I had explored, including the macrobiotic diet and yoga. I then shared with them my first, unsuccessful experience with T'ai Chi.

Sister Antonia assured me that T'ai Chi Chih was not a martial art and was indeed gentle. She then contrasted T'ai Chi Chih with yoga by explaining that it was a meditation practice based not on breathing but on movements that balanced yin and yang. The goal was to let the body heal itself during the pauses – the silence – between the moves.

Sister Antonia encouraged me to start slowly. As she explained the first movement – a rocking motion – she gave each of us the option to execute the move from a seated position rather than standing, a gentle compromise that reminded me of the careful methods of my yoga instructor Michelle Kouri. By modifying the exercises to make them easier, I managed to participate in the entire forty-five-minute class and drove home from my first day of T'ai Chi Chih feeling energized rather than frustrated or deficient.

The class continued to be held in the hospital's chapel, which I soon began to appreciate as an uncannily beautiful site for our healing work. Sunlight streamed through the stained glass windows on clear days, creating patterns of purple, red, yellow, and green on the floor. As we all moved in unison in such a nurturing, peaceful setting, I felt blessed to be part of a group – such a stark contrast to all of the time I had spent alone during my recovery.

Sister Antonia waxed poetic about grounding at one of our morning sessions, directing our awareness to our feet. "Take time when you walk down the street to think about your feet," she said.

I did as she suggested and found that her advice made a substantial difference in how I felt as I moved. The sensation was one of coming out of my head and into my body, an act that I found challenging, to say the least. Fortunately, I found the movements of T'ai Chi Chih to be simple and beautiful, so it made the hard work pleasurable.

After completing the eight-week course, I continued to practice T'ai Chi Chih and yoga at home every morning, and the combination of the two disciplines further increased my awareness of the relationship between physical, emotional, and spiritual healing. T'ai Chi Chih gave me a dose of humility as well, reminding me that, despite how far I'd gone and despite how much work I'd already put in, I still had a long way to go as far as my healing was concerned. I was learning, slowly and incrementally, to become a whole person, which for me largely meant resisting the tyranny of my mind.

My neighbor Joan, a widower and like me a former nurse, gave me the perfect opportunity to do exactly that when she invited me to join her for her bimonthly pilgrimage to the Florida coast, where she owned a beach house. I had often looked after Joan's cat – the cat that had arrived on my doorstep the morning after my father had passed away – during her past excursions, and she had reciprocated by seeing me through some of the worst moments of my illness. She made a perfect vacation partner, and we relished the opportunity to enjoy each other's company in better circumstances. She was interested in my healing transformation and listened patiently as I described the road I'd taken since languishing on death's door.

While at her beach house I practiced my T'ai Chi Chih exercises by the ocean each morning. The sound of the surf made for a perfect backdrop, and I let myself sink into the serenity of each movement.

Several fishermen asked me what I was doing when I went out at dawn to practice the first morning, and I gave them a brief explanation of T'ai Chi Chih, encouraging them to try it with me. Skeptical, they asked what it could do for them if they tried.

"Well," I responded, "it might improve your fishing!"

A couple of the older fellows tried the rocking motion with me, and on the next day a couple more salty and weathered men joined me. By the last day of my vacation, there were fourteen of us down there on the beach.

This, I realized, was what it meant to live in the present, to know each moment as an eternity.

§§

As soon as I had returned from Florida, I signed up for another eight weeks of T'ai Chi Chih classes, and after completing the series, I told Sister Antonia I wanted to learn how to teach the practice. She encouraged me but also counseled that, if I wanted to be ready for the accreditation class that would come the following May, I would have to practice every single day.

I felt a strong desire to teach and immediately threw myself into a rigorous preparation program, but it didn't take long to realize that I just didn't have the coordination or balance yet that I would need to meet the deadline. So I decided to set a goal for accreditation for May of 1995, which would give me roughly one and a half years to prepare myself. This would also give me time to resurrect my real estate career, which I had been unable to pursue while ill.

§§

As I started to ramp up my business again, I was surprised to find that I was bringing a new energy to the work. Yoga, meditation, and T'ai Chi Chih all helped me approach the day-to-day challenges of real estate in a fundamentally new way. When clients or coworkers responded irrationally to situations, I didn't absorb their emotions. Instead, I found myself able to respond – most of the time, anyway – in a calm, measured way. My daily routine kept me grounded, and I paid dearly when I strayed from it for more than a day or two. Not only would I experience more stress; I could literally feel it in the hardness of my skin.

It took discipline to stay centered, to stay true to myself. I often thought of my vacation in Florida and my epiphany while practicing T'ai Chi Chih with the fishermen down on the beach. My recurring dream didn't have to be about drowning. It could be about learning to live all over again.

⌘ 21 ⌘

In May of 1994, part of a tooth on the bottom right side of my mouth broke off while I was eating. My first reaction was to worry. Scleroderma often causes teeth to break or fall out because it shrinks the gums. Was I truly on the road back? Or was my broken tooth an ominous sign of things to come?

I immediately made an appointment with a dentist to get some advice, and when I saw him he assured me he could save the tooth by doing a root canal. However, he had found an abscess under the tooth and informed me that he couldn't begin the root canal until the infection cleared. I left his office with a two-week prescription for antibiotics and plenty of time to think about his recommendation.

My only experience with a root canal dated back to the 1970s, when a dentist had also recommended one for one of my teeth. The offending tooth had cracked during the procedure, forcing the dentist to extract it instead. I couldn't help wondering if that might happen again.

I also questioned the safety of root canal work in general. I had read literature over the years that suggested some people experienced long-term health problems as a result of the procedure. I thought back to my lone childhood visit to the dentist – the one that ended with my sister Evelyn and me sneaking out of the dispensary after receiving a shot each of Novocain – and realized as an adult I felt grateful for dental care but was also open to other options, including unconventional ones; my experience with healing so far had shown me that anything was possible.

I had barely begun to investigate my options when I received a flyer in the mail advertising a holistic medicine seminar. The list of speakers included Dr. Tom Haffner, DDS, a dentist who practiced in Upper Saddle River, a town about thirty minutes by car from my house. Intrigued, I called Dr. Haffner's office and made an appointment to get a second opinion on my tooth.

Dr. Haffner, who headed up New Jersey's Holistic Society, was a tall man whose son also practiced dentistry and worked in his clinic. Dr. Haffner was famous for leaving his patients reclining, mouths open wide, while he drove off to the local deli for a sandwich. Something about him made it impossible for anyone to be mad at him. "It was an emergency," he would say when confronted.

At my first meeting with him, he x-rayed my teeth and after studying the x-rays confirmed my dentist's diagnosis.

"Yes," he said, "there's an abscess under the broken tooth. But what happened to your upper palate?"

I told him the roof of my mouth was deformed because of my illness and that I had subsisted on a liquefied diet for several years. Now that I had started to eat solid food again, I explained, the roof of my mouth had narrowed so much that food often got stuck there when I ate.

Dr. Haffner nodded as I laid out my problems in detail – he would later show me a handful of exercises to help my tongue make contact with the roof of my mouth – and then recommended that I forgo the root canal and have the broken tooth extracted instead.

With that solved, Dr. Haffner asked me if I had ever heard of Crosatt Therapy. When I answered no, he explained that it was a form of orthodontics for children and adults that corrected the bite. In my case, he told me, it could help ease the overcrowding of my lower teeth and fill in the space made when he extracted the tooth. It would involve installing a removable metal apparatus in my mouth, which, if it worked correctly, would move the bones of my skull to improve the problems with my bite and my palate.

I left Dr. Haffner's office thinking the procedure seemed a little far-fetched. Moreover, I had reservations about proceeding with a tooth extraction. I didn't want to subject my face and head – not to mention my psyche – to the trauma of an extraction after I had already endured so much pain from scleroderma. Would Crosatt Therapy induce new problems?

I brought my quandary to Dr. Whitman, who was up front as always in his response.

"It could trigger inflammation," he said matter-of-factly, "and your face might blow up like a balloon. But it's your call."

After debating the pros and cons, I finally decided to make an appointment with Dr. Haffner to have the tooth extracted. The surgery, to my surprise and relief, was painless. I didn't even experience soreness the following day. The extraction went so smoothly, in fact, that I decided to proceed with the Crosatt Therapy.

Dr. Haffner fitted me with a wire contraption, which he popped onto my back teeth. It was no small feat, considering I still had numbness in my face and still had difficulty opening my mouth.

I watched for any adverse reactions in the ensuing days after the procedure. None came. My mouth felt a bit like a highway under construction, but I escaped without swelling, pain, or increased numbness.

Just a few weeks into wearing the apparatus, I noticed a subtle widening in my nose and the area around it. After a few months, other people began noticing that my face looked different, commenting that it was no longer so narrow and actually looked more . . . normal.

Their comments were music to my ears. When a few more months went by and the bones around my eyes and mouth began to open up, I knew the therapy was making a difference.

⚭

I continued to hone my T'ai Chi Chih skills, meanwhile, practicing every day and slowly working toward accreditation, with Sister Antonia mentoring me every step of the way. My coordination had improved greatly in the last year, although I probably wasn't Sister Antonia's easiest student. I often wondered if I was responsible for turning her hair an even brighter shade of snow-white.

Perhaps my biggest hurdle was physical discomfort. Sometimes as I practiced T'ai Chi Chih, pain would surface in the form of a burning sensation in my face. At other times the pain migrated to the right side of my head or my shoulder. I wondered if the discomfort meant that I was practicing improperly. Worse still, I wondered if the practice wasn't working for me. As I tried to sort through my difficulties, I came across an article on T'ai Chi Chih that suggested my problems with discomfort could be traced to resistance. I was resisting the integration of yin and yang.

As I learned to see the pain as an expression of my resistance, I found myself practicing with a more relaxed mind and I let my awareness shift to whatever part of my body was tense. The more I relaxed into the moves and into the rest period – the silence – between the moves where the yin and yang integrated, the more I learned how to let go. I became convinced as my resistance gradually waned that my body had been crying out for this type of energy work for years. The T'ai Chi Chih exercises gave me a sense of serenity and peace. When my energy flowed freely, I felt as if the movements were occurring without any effort from me. I was learning to trust myself and the universe.

I finally mastered T'ai Chi Chih and became an accredited teacher in May of 1995, just as I had hoped. The last portion of my training program took place at the Carmel Retreat Center in Mahwah, New Jersey, where the students and instructors spent a week together in retreat. We practiced for two hours every morning, then met for four hours of class work each evening. The instructors, including Sister Antonia, nurtured us and made us feel at ease.

One instructor, Steve Ridley, emphasized that we needed understanding and skill for accreditation, not perfection. Steve, who also introduced us to other forms of energy work, including the 18-form Qi Gong, was one of the most relaxed persons I'd ever met. Every movement, every lesson he imparted, was a demonstration in letting go.

I felt so close to him and the other instructors as well as my fellow students that I hated leaving when the week finally came to an end. We had begun to learn, as Steve put it, to "embrace ourselves as the embodied essence."

ᘒᘒ

It was time, once again, to measure my progress. A month had gone by since my T'ai Chi Chih accreditation, and as I visited Dr. Whitman to review the results from my latest blood work, I couldn't help marveling at how far I'd come. My hands looked perfectly normal again, as did my feet. I stood straight and tall. I no longer suffered the debilitating attacks courtesy of Raynaud's phenomenon. And my skin, rock-hard and taut as a drum for so long, appeared healthy and supple.

Nearly seven years had passed since Dr. Whitman had diagnosed my illness and floored me with his dire prognosis, and as my trusted doctor sat across from me and reviewed my bulging file, a look of wry disbelief spread across his face.

"It looks like right now you're clear of scleroderma," he said in his typically understated fashion.

Dr. Whitman had never been one to waste words. Nor was he the demonstrative type. But I didn't need a congratulatory speech. I felt like I had just won a million dollars – more than that. A triumphant feeling surged through me, followed quickly by a wave of gratitude. I had endured an incredible journey, with more than its share of ups and downs. And scleroderma, my teacher, had finally bid farewell.

Until that moment it had been easy to second-guess my recovery. But it was right there in my blood work. As of that day in June 1995, my ANA count had fallen to zero, which indicated a complete remission.

"When I think back to the first day I saw you," Dr. Whitman mused, "I can't believe you recovered. This is truly a miracle."

Indeed it was. But the miracle needed several more months to come to complete fruition. My nightly prayer – that I might someday look in the mirror and see my face again, instead of the face of scleroderma – came true the following year as I finished Crosatt Therapy. When Dr. Haffner had originally proposed the unorthodox treatment, he hadn't said anything about reshaping my face. He had confined his goals to expanding my palate and repairing my bite so I could eat and digest my food more efficiently. But by 1996, my palate had opened up beautifully, my chin and face had widened, and I looked like . . . me.

৩৫ 22 ৩৫

When I first came to the United States, people often asked me, "Has anyone ever told you how much you look like Katherine Hepburn?"

"Katherine who?" was usually my response.

We didn't see too many movies while growing up in Ireland, and I had never heard of the famous American actress. As luck would have it, one day I had the great pleasure of meeting her when she came to visit a sick friend at the hospital where I worked. She had aged significantly by then, and I thought, *Oh, my God, I don't look like her!* But later I saw pictures of her during her heyday, and I thought that perhaps there was a resemblance between us.

When I was ill and disfigured by scleroderma, *nobody* told me I looked like Katherine Hepburn. I knew I had come full circle when, a few years after being declared in full remission, I was getting out of my car to show a house to some clients and they said, "Oh, my Lord! Has anyone ever told you how much you look like Katherine Hepburn?" They couldn't see any traces in my face of what I'd been through.

Would that all victims of scleroderma could enjoy a similar experience! But the stark truth remains: few beat the illness; most take it with them to the grave. More accurate, most die an early death, thanks to the disease.

᭰᭰

Years earlier, close to the peak of my illness, I had gone to a client's home in my neighborhood to put together a complimentary market analysis (CMA). My hands were giving me grief at the time, and I was barely holding it together. But I tried to fake it long enough to complete the walk-through of the house and then return with an analysis the next day for the client, a sixty-year-old woman who, along with her husband, wanted to find out what her home was worth on the market.

Unfortunately, I was running a fever and feeling awful the next day and couldn't make good on my promise, so I asked a coworker to finish the CMA for me and deliver it to the client. My coworker obliged and told the woman that I had the flu.

I didn't hear back from the woman until St. Patrick's Day arrived a few days later. I was sick once again and in bed when the doorbell rang. I panicked at the sound, momentarily wishing the floor would open up and swallow me. Finally I stirred up enough courage to trudge downstairs to the front door and open it. Standing there was the sixty-year-old woman I had just visited a few days ago. She smiled and handed me a tiny pot of shamrocks.

"Happy Saint Patrick's Day," she said cheerfully.

I drooled and choked on my answer, barely able to respond to her. Likewise, it was all I could do to grasp the tiny pot of shamrocks with my swollen hands.

I was overcome with shame – shame that I had wasted away to such a frightening degree and shame that anyone, least of all a client and a neighbor, had seen me in my wretched state. She left abruptly, and I didn't hear back from her for some time.

As the weeks and months wore on and I began to walk around the neighborhood lake as part of my recovery, I occasionally ran into the woman with the shamrocks.

"Hi, Maureen!" she would say cheerfully. "How are you?"

I usually responded in the affirmative: "Fine, thanks." I never offered an explanation for that day, other than to say that I had had the flu. And she never pressed the issue.

We kept in contact off and on for the next several years, with my updating her on the conditions of the local real estate market whenever she queried me.

Finally, after I had been in remission for quite some time, she called me one night on the telephone. "Maureen," she said, "we're ready to sell our house, and we're thinking of choosing you to put it on the market."

I was happy to assist her and returned to her home to put together another market analysis. She was sitting across the table from me when we were all finished and said, "Maureen, I have a question for you. How did you overcome your scleroderma?"

I was floored. She had known all along.

"Tell me," I said in amazement, "how did you know what I had?"

As she gazed silently at me, her eyes filled with tears. "My beautiful daughter died from it," she finally said. "The night you were first here, I knew that you had the disease. You didn't say anything, and I knew it was difficult for you even to talk. That morning at the door, I saw my daughter in you."

I remembered she had left abruptly the day she had brought me the tiny pot of shamrocks.

"My daughter died when she was twenty-six," she explained. "I saw her hands and I saw her face all over again on your doorstep. My husband never wanted to talk about the disease. He never wanted me to get involved with any of the foundations."

I nodded knowingly, having suffered through various stages of denial and anger myself. After I told her my story, she urged me to share my healing process with the public, especially with others who suffered with scleroderma.

❦

When I had been sick myself, I would have given anything to hear that just one person had gone into remission and, perhaps most important to me, fully reversed the disfigurement from the disease.

So I thought hard about my client's request. My heart went out to those suffering from scleroderma, but I was hesitant to undertake the mission of sharing my healing process. I feared going public with my story might be the death of my privacy. I also knew that by telling my story I would have to revisit the pain of the ordeal, and I couldn't quite face reliving the experience. Finally, I knew that, although I had healed, I hadn't discovered a magic bullet that could cure others. I wasn't even sure whether or not I had discovered a particular combination of therapies that could cure anybody but me.

A few weeks after my conversation with my client, a reporter from The *Herald News*, our town paper, called to ask about my recovery. I suspected my client had given the reporter my name, so I invited him into my home for an interview. His wonderful piece appeared in print in early January of 1996.

Later that year, a larger newspaper, The *Bergen Record*, featured a piece on my recovery. Then *Women's World* magazine picked up the story and ran an article, which first appeared on newsstands at the end of December. I didn't know much about *Women's World* at the time. In fact, I assumed it had a rather small circulation, so I wasn't prepared for the deluge of responses coming my way.

On New Year's Day, 1997, my home phone rang off the hook. It continued to do so – twenty-four hours a day – for several weeks. People from all over the world called to find out more details about my healing process. Some of them had suffered from systemic sclerosis for years, while others had just received a diagnosis.

I talked to everyone who called, then talked to some of them again over the following weeks. Many called a second or third time, asking for more information about the alternative therapies I had tried because their doctors doubted my credibility and the efficacy of my unconventional treatment.

Three years later, *Extra TV* produced a segment about my story, and after it aired I could barely keep up with the inquiries I received. As phone calls and e-mails poured in, people pressed hard for an answer to the most vexing question of all: What was the one thing you did to reverse your disease?

Although I wished I could deliver the magic bullet they hoped to find, I didn't want simply to tell people what they wanted to hear.

Instead, I explained that my recovery was characterized by several equally important factors.

The first was excellent medical care. Yes, it had taken what felt like forever to hunt down a proper diagnosis, but I found in Dr. Whitman a caring, qualified professional, someone who was willing to treat me like a partner throughout my recovery, someone who was open to unconventional ideas and treatments.

The second was unflinching determination. I had many, many low moments. Moments where all felt lost, where all I wanted to do was escape my body and the misery it provoked. But I survived every blow scleroderma dealt me and vowed to keep on fighting. Countless studies warned the same thing: I was traveling a one-way road with no hope of turning back. But I refused to take that road.

The third was wholehearted trial and error of drugs, nutritional programs, herbs, and physical therapies. Despite my fears, and despite the skepticism of others, I tried anything I thought held promise. The bedrock of my treatment, of course, was conventional care, specifically the somewhat radical antibiotic therapy. But through it all I learned to trust my body and recognize my instincts. As mentioned above, I was lucky to work with Dr. Whitman, who didn't force me to choose between types of care but let me explore for myself what was available to me.

This leads to the fourth aspect of my recovery, which was the courage to harness intuition as my guide. Throughout life we are conditioned to trust the experts, to hand our care over to more qualified professionals. But most often the person who knows best what will heal you is . . . you. It took me a while, but I learned how to sit still long enough to listen to the wisdom within.

Finally, I had faith. Faith in myself. Faith in my spirit. Though disenchanted with the Catholic religion, I still believed in the power of prayer and in the power of the human mind. When it seemed everything – including my own body – wanted me dead, I *willed* myself to health. I logged countless hours meditating, praying, stretching, and exercising, and I conditioned my mind to want only one thing: total remission.

In the end, my healing was an exercise in metamorphosis – an acknowledgement of personal power, of the power to create. But my metamorphosis didn't happen overnight. It emerged only after a long and arduous process. I would never want to take that journey again, but I would never part with the lessons scleroderma taught me. I learned to embrace the healing wisdom of my body, that inscrutable mystery, which I somehow – awkwardly, haphazardly, and often unwittingly – penetrated by thinking with my heart and galvanizing my will.

I hope such an insight is my legacy. I'd like to think that someday, even after I'm long gone, someone will come across my story and discover the power to heal. Whether that someone is suffering from scleroderma, cancer, or obesity – it doesn't matter. All that matters is that we recognize the power hidden in all of us to remake the world.

❧ Epilogue ❧

Best-selling author and medical doctor Bernie Siegel describes disease as "a call to change." It certainly was for me. When I became ill, I felt as if the world had come to an end, as if it had moved on and left me behind. I had nowhere to go.

But scleroderma taught me that indeed I did have a place to go. The place was deep within me, and in the years that followed, as I struggled to regain my health and my beauty, I realized that my essence – that part of me buried deep inside – already knew the road back to full recovery. Paradoxically, when I finally let go of worrying about my disfigured face and my contorted hands, when I finally let go of the anger and the hurt and the pain that had accumulated over a lifetime of ups and downs, I found relief and recovery.

We manufacture two faces: one for the outside world and one we keep hidden inside. The inner one is who we truly are. It deserves to shine. Scleroderma was all about self-protection and control. As I slowly healed, I found myself opening like a flower blooming in the warm spring air. My hunched body straightened. My hands uncurled. Layer after protective layer fell away as I shed a belief system that no longer served me and rebuilt one that spoke to my true self.

My rebirth is not perfect. Nor is it complete. It is an ongoing process. One that moves forward in fits and starts. Although I am in remission from scleroderma, I continue to nurture my health. In particular, I still take time for myself every morning. I continue a daily routine which includes T'ai Chi Chih and meditation. In fact, if I leave the house in the morning without doing my routine, I feel as if I haven't put my shoes on.

My newfound health feels like liberation. I can look in the mirror each day without seeing scleroderma staring back at me. I can scrape the ice off my car's windshield on a frosty winter morning without suffering an attack of Raynaud's phenomenon. These days I have boundless energy. I hardly ever get sick.

But I'm not so removed from my former life that I can't remember what it felt like to live with a death sentence. My emotions often get the best of me when I attend the funeral of someone who has died of scleroderma because I can't help but identify with that person. I know all too well what it was like for them in their final days.

I worry, too, for those among the living who still suffer with the disease. Who will they turn to? Who will champion their cause? If, like me, they set out to heal themselves, they will be awfully vulnerable to charlatans who prey on the desperate. I hope they find the courage to try anything – and to toss whatever doesn't work.

I still get dozens of calls and e-mails each month from sufferers of scleroderma. Often they are poor or lack adequate health insurance. I try to give them a sliver of hope, the sort of hope that empowered me.

I doubt I'm the only person ever to recover completely from the disfigurement of scleroderma, but I know my story is rare. Rarer still is how complete and life-changing my metamorphosis has been. I look better now than I did when I was forty.

In the past two years, I have learned a new form of meditation called Pan Gu Qigong, which I find immensely beneficial. Pan Gu Qigong integrates the energy of the sun and the moon to regenerate the body and spirit. When I practice its movements, I can feel energy surge through my body.

I still occasionally listen to Depak Chopra's tape, which has never lost its value for me. I have learned to relish my moments alone. My experience with scleroderma taught me that I desperately need that quiet time for myself every day. If I don't make time for meditating and exercising, my body reminds me in short order what it needs. I discovered someone within me, someone buried for most of my life, and I'm not about to let her go.

My husband, Bob, and I continued to live together under the same roof after our divorce for another ten years before we parted as good friends. I felt so many strong emotions – anger, abandonment – toward him during my illness. Now I realize he gave what he could in the only way he could. As I look back at our marriage, I realize we were meant to be together, if only briefly, and we learned much from each other. I wish him well.

My brother Chris passed away just before Christmas in 2003, from prostate cancer. It was difficult to lose a sibling and another member of my family, and I still miss him. Sometimes on my way from work in the morning I talk to him. But I found solace in the fact that he had been released from his body. He's resting comfortably somewhere else now. I know he is happy.

Donna Powel, my tall redheaded friend with the unforgettable laugh, eventually moved to sunny Florida. We still keep in touch, and to this day I still ponder a little kernel of wisdom she shared with me on more than one occasion: be patient. She knew as well as I did that patience often eluded me. I'd like to think I've since learned how to wait for the future to come – and how to sit quietly with myself in the interim. But that kind of serenity doesn't come easily to me. Nor, I suspect, to anyone.

My beloved Westies, meanwhile, have all since passed away. McDuff lived to a ripe old seventeen years of age. A wonderful dog, he spent most of his years sitting in my lap, whether I was on the phone, entertaining a visitor, or not feeling well. His habit of jumping into my lap and staring deeply into my eyes was usually successful in getting him what he deserved: my attention. Kerry died of lymphosarcoma at age twelve. Taidy, a head-shy dog we rescued from an abusive situation, only made it to ten before succumbing to a host of ailments, including diabetes and lung cancer.

I now have two new companions: a cairn terrier named Busy and a Bichon named Tess, who I adopted from a shelter. I will never forget my Westies, whose photographs still grace the refrigerator. They were only dogs, some might argue, but they were there with me during my lowest moments. When scleroderma brought me to my knees, I found loving canine eyes staring back at me. They taught me what I already knew: that humanity cuts across the biological divide.

I still meet for regular checkups with Dr. Whitman, who has since become a great believer in nutrition and the vital role it plays in healing.

"I don't know if the macrobiotic diet is the answer," he told me recently. "It made you so emaciated. But certainly the change in your diet, along with antibiotic therapy, seems to have been an essential ingredient in making you well again." At the time of this writing, Dr. Whitman suggests the macrobiotic diet to some of his scleroderma patients.

These days, I keep a busy schedule. I work part-time in my real estate business and have returned part-time to private duty nursing as well, but I always make time to go home for a healthy lunch. I don't follow the macrobiotic diet religiously anymore. But I still subscribe to macrobiotic principles for the most part. I eat no meat, aside from a very occasional piece of fish. I live on salads, grains, and legumes, and sometimes I get additional protein from an egg or a piece of cheese made from goat's milk. I no longer sleep on a magnetic bed and only rarely take herbal supplements.

I continue to trust myself and the universe, and I know that I have nothing to fear. The disease that once controlled my life has no power over me now. By forcing me to change, scleroderma gave me my freedom – and a place to go.